PROSTAGLANDINS AND IMMUNITY

PROSTAGLANDINS, LEUKOTRIENES, AND CANCER

Series Editors: Kenneth V. Honn and Lawrence J. Marnett
Wayne State University School of Medicine
Detroit, Michigan

W.E.M. Lands, ed.: Biochemistry of Arachidonic Acid Metabolism. 1985. ISBN 0-89838-717-5.

L.J. Marnett, ed.: Arachidonic Acid Metabolism and Tumor Initiation. 1985. ISBN 0-89838-729-9.

S.M. Fischer and T.J. Slaga, eds.: Arachidonic Acid Metabolism and Tumor Promotion. 1985. ISBN 0-89838-724-8.

J.S. Goodwin, ed.: Prostaglandins and Immunity. 1985. ISBN 0-89838-723-X.

PROSTAGLANDINS AND IMMUNITY

edited by

J.S. Goodwin
University of New Mexico
School of Medicine

Martinus Nijhoff Publishing
a member of the Kluwer Academic Publishers Group
Boston/Dordrecht/Lancaster

Distributors for North America:
Kluwer Academic Publishers
190 Old Derby Street
Hingham, MA 02043

Distributors for all other countries:
Kluwer Academic Publishers Group
Distribution Centre
P.O. Box 322
3300 AH Dordrecht
The Netherlands

Library of Congress Cataloging in Publication Data

Main entry under title:

Prostaglandins and immunity.

(Prostaglandins, leukotrienes, and cancer)
Includes bibliographies and index.
1. Immune response—Regulation. 2. Prostaglandins.
3. Arachidonic acid—Metabolism. 4. Immunopharmacology.
I. Goodwin, James S., 1945- . II. Series.
[DNLM: 1. Prostaglandins—immunology. QU 90 P967135]
QR186.P76 1985 616.07'9 85-4989
ISBN 0-89838-723-X

Printed in the United States of America

CONTENTS

ABRAMSON, S., Division of Rheumatology, Department of Medicine, New York University Medical Center, 550 First Avenue, New York, NY 10016, U.S.A.

ALDIGIER, J.C., Immunologie and Biochemistry Research Unit, School of Medicine, 2 rue du Dr. Marcland, 87032 Limoges Cedex, France.

CEUPPENS, J.L., Klinische Immunologie, Katholieke Universiteit Leuven, Kapucijnenvoer 33, 3000 Leuven, Belgium.

CHIRIGOS, M.A., Immunopharmacology Section, Biological Therapeutics Branch, Biological Response Modifiers Program, National Cancer Institute, Frederick Cancer Research Facility, Frederick, MD 21701, U.S.A.

DROLLER, M.J., James Buchanan Brady Urological Institute, The Johns Hopkins Hospital, Baltimore, MD 21205, U.S.A.

DURANDY, A., Institut National de la Santé et de la Recherche Médicale, Groupe de Recherches d'Immunologie et de Rhumatologie Pédiatriques, Hôpital des Enfants Malades, 149 Rue de Sèvres, 75743 Paris Cedex 15, France.

FANTONE, J.C., Department of Pathology, University of Michigan School of Medicine, Ann Arbor, MI 48109, U.S.A.

FISCHER, A., Institut National de la Santé et de la Recherche Médicale, Groupe de Recherches d'Immunologie et de Rhumatologie Pédiatriques, Hôpital des Enfants Malades, 149 Rue de Sèvres, 75743 Paris Cedex 15, France.

GOODWIN, J.S., Division of Gerontology, Department of Medicine, University of New Mexico School of Medicine, Albuquerque, NM 87131, U.S.A.

GRISCELLI, C., Institut National de la Santé et de la Recherche Médicale, Groupe de Recherches d'Immunologie et de Rhumatologie Pédiatriques, Hôpital des Enfants Malades, 149 Rue de Sèvres, 75743 Paris Cedex 15, France.

GUALDE, N., Immunologie and Biochemistry Research Unit, School of Medicine, 2 rue du Dr. Marcland, 87032 Limoges Cedex, France.

HARTUNG, K., Immunopharmacology Section, Biological Therapeutics Branch, Biological Response Modifiers Program, National Cancer Institute, Frederick Cancer Research Facility, Frederick, MD 21701, U.S.A.

KORCHAK, H.M., Division of Rheumatology, Department of Medicine, New York University Medical Center, 550 First Avenue, New York, NY 10016, U.S.A.

KUNKEL, S., Department of Pathology, University of Michigan School of Medicine, Ann Arbor, MI 48109, U.S.A.

LE DEIST, F., Institut National de la Santé et de la Recherche Médicale, Groupe de Recherches d'Immunologie et de Rhumatologie Pédiatriques, Hôpital des Enfants Malades, 149 Rue de Sèvres, 75743 Paris Cedex 15, France.

MEXMAIN, S., Immunologie and Biochemistry Research Unit, School of Medicine, 2 rue du Dr. Marcland, 87032 Limoges Cedex, France.

ROGERS, T.J., Department of Microbiology and Immunology, Temple University School of Medicine, Philadelphia, PA 19140, U.S.A.

SCHLICK, E., Lymphokines Section, Laboratory of Molecular Immunoregulation, Biological Response Modifiers Program, National Cancer Institute, Frederick Cancer Research Facility, Frederick, MD 21701, U.S.A.

ZURIER, R.B., Rheumatology Section, Department of Medicine, University of Pennsylvania School of Medicine, 3400 Spruce Street, Philadelphia, PA 19104, U.S.A.

FOREWORD

Prostaglandins, Leukotrienes, and Cancer is a multi-volume series that will focus on an emerging area of cancer research. In 1968, R.H. Williams first reported that elevated prostaglandin levels are present in human medullary carcinoma. Since that time, the concept that arachidonic acid metabolites may be involved in cancer has expanded to include every aspect of the disease from cell transformation through metastasis.

Prostaglandins and leukotrienes are generic terms used to describe a family of bioactive lipids produced from unsaturated fatty acids (principally from arachidonic acid) via the cyclooxygenase and lipoxygenase pathways, respectively. Cyclooxygenase products consist of diverse products such as prostaglandin E_2 (PGE_2), prostacyclin (PGI_2) and thromboxane A_2 (TXA_2), whereas lipoxygenase products consist of hydroperoxy fatty acids and mono-, di- and tri-hydroxy acids including leukotrienes. The precursor fatty acids for the cyclooxygenase and lipoxygenase pathways are present in cellular phospholipids. This finding established an important control point in their biosynthesis—the release of substrate. This occurs in response to numerous stimuli that act at the cell surface. Dr. Bengt Samuelsson's extensive study of the metabolism of prostaglandins indicated that they are rapidly inactivated on a single pass through pulmonary circulation. Thus, they cannot act as circulating hormones and appear to be made on demand in or in the vicinity of target tissues leading to the concept that prostaglandins are local hormones or autocoids.

Altered production, qualitative and/or quantitative, of prostaglandins and leukotrienes has been implicated in the development of a number of disease states (e.g., atherosclerosis, inflammatory diseases, asthma). Evidence has been accumulating in the literature suggesting that prostaglandins and leukotrienes may stimulate or inhibit various steps in the complex etiology of cancer, i.e., steps in the progression from a transformed cell to a metastatic tumor. The initial volumes in this series will examine the roles of prostaglandins and leukotrienes in tumor initiation, tumor promotion, tumor cell growth and differentiation, tumor immunity, tumor metastasis and cancer therapy. We hope as this field of cancer research develops that this series, Prostaglandins, Leukotrienes, and Cancer, will provide a forum within the framework of current evidence for the synthesis of new hypotheses and discussion of controversial issues.

Kenneth V. Honn
Lawrence J. Marnett

PREFACE

My goal in compiling this volume is to produce a comprehensive review of current knowledge of the role of arachidonic acid metabolites on immune function. To this end I have invited investigators who have been pursuing various aspects of this issue to summarize their own work and the relevant work from other laboratories on specific topics in this general area. I have assumed that the major audience for this book will come from three sources. First, immunopharmacologists, whether or not they are specifically working in the area of arachidonic acid metabolites, may find this a useful summary of that area of immunopharmacology dealing with manipulations of arachidonic acid metabolism. Second, any investigator involved in piecing together the roles for the various arachidonic acid metabolites in any physiologic system--renal, endocrine, cardiovascular, etc.--may find that a review of analogous work in the immune system may suggest new methods of approach in his or her specific area. Finally, immunologists interested in the endogenous regulation of the immune response should find here a compilation of one aspect of that regulation by the local hormones derived from arachidonic acid. My assumptions about the audience have influenced the selection of material and also the manner of presentation chosen by the individual contributors. We have not assumed, for example, that the reader is necessarily an immunologist or is intimately familiar with arachidonic acid metabolism.

One problem with volumes comprised of papers from different laboratories about different aspects of one issue is that there tends to be some overlap among the chapters. A quick glance through the bibliographies to the chapters in this book will reveal many references that pop up repeatedly. There is essentially no way to avoid this while still allowing each chapter to stand by itself. It is necessary for each investigator to put his or her work in context, and the context, while varying in emphasis from chapter to chapter, is still quite similar for all the contributions to this book.

It almost goes without saying that arachidonic acid metabolism is a rapidly evolving field. Terms that were coined quite recently, like leukotrienes, have found their way into everyday scientific and medical parlance. A simplified scheme of arachidonic acid metabolism is presented in Figure 1. It is important to realize that the great mass of lipoxygenase metabolites have not yet been identified; nor, obviously, have their biologic roles been characterized. On the other hand, most stable cyclooxygenase products have been available for study for more than a decade. Accordingly, quite a bit more is known about the physiologic roles of these products, and this advantage is reflected in the greater space in this volume devoted to cyclooxygenase rather than lipoxygenase products. Because phospholipase A_2 activation, the first step in arachidonic acid metabolism, is as ubiquitous a response to stimuli as is adenylate cyclase activation, it is safe to assume that the eventual list of biologic actions of the leukotrienes and other lipoxygenase metabolites of arachidonic acid will be considerably longer than it is today.

One line of evidence suggesting critical roles for lipoxygenase products in immune function comes from the powerful immunomodulating properties of corticosteroids. It would appear that many and perhaps all of the physiologic and pharmacologic effects of corticosteroids are secondary to inhibition of phospholipase A_2 inhibition. In 1977, Gryglewski et al. (1) and several other groups (2-4) showed that steroids inhibit the release of arachidonic acid from membrane phospholipids and proposed that the anti-inflammatory activity of steroids is due to this action. The schema of arachidonic acid metabolism in Figure 1 allows us to consider the possibility that many of the pharmacologic and physiologic actions of steroids are indeed via inhibition of arachidonic acid release from membrane

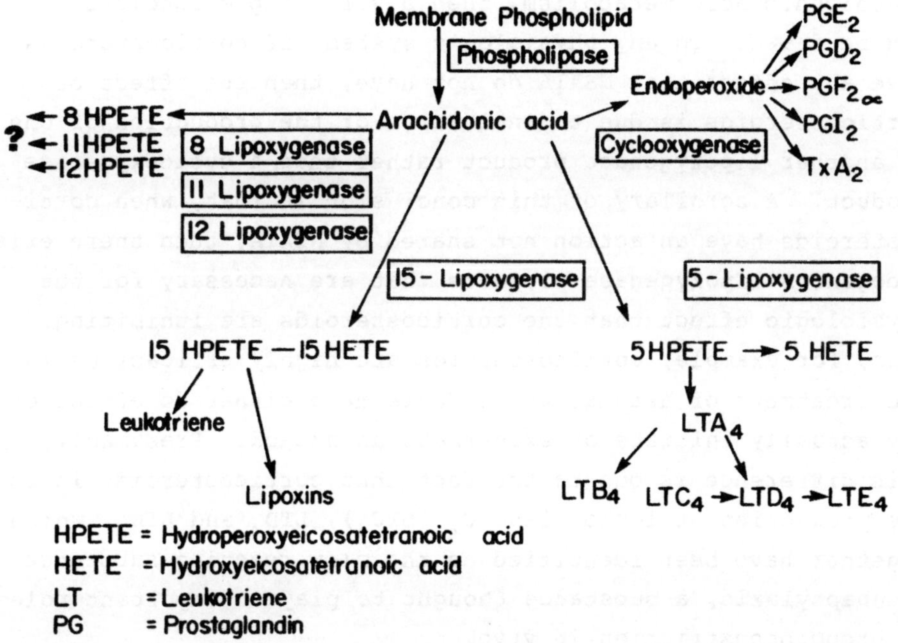

FIGURE 1. Somewhat simplified schema of arachidonic acid metabolism.

phospholipid. Steroids would then inhibit both cyclooxygenase and lipoxygenase products while non-steroidal anti-inflammatory agents (NSAIA) inhibit only cyclooxygenase products. Clearly, the evidence supporting this concept has grown considerably over the past few years. Danon and Assouline showed that RNA and protein synthesis is required in order for steroids to inhibit prostaglandin (PG) production (5). In 1979 and 1980, Flower and his associates in England and Hirata, Axelrod and their coworkers at the NIH identified a phospholipase A_2-inhibitory glycoprotein, termed macrocortin or lipomodulin, synthesized and released by cells upon exposure to corticosteroid (6-8). Recent evidence suggests that macrocortin, with an estimated molecular weight of ~40,000, is a polymer or aggregate of lipomodulin, with a molecular weight of ~14,000.

If, indeed, the pharmacologic effects of corticosteroids are due to inhibition of phospholipase A_2, thereby inhibiting arachidonic acid metabolism, then a very simple conclusion can be drawn: in any physiologic system, if corticosteroids have any effect that NSAIA do not have, then the effect of corticosteroids is due to inhibition of the production of one or another lipoxygenase product rather than a cyclooxygenase product. A corollary of this conclusion is that, when corticosteroids have an action not shared by NSAIA, then there exist endogenous lipoxygenase products that are necessary for the physiologic effect that the corticosteroids are inhibiting. Thus, for example, corticosteroids are highly efficacious in the treatment of asthma, while NSAIA have either no effect or may actually initiate or exacerbate an attack. Presumably, this difference is due to the fact that corticosteroids inhibit the production of leukotriene C_4 (LTC_4), LTD_4 and LTE_4, which together have been identified as the slow reacting substance of anaphylaxis, a substance thought to play an important role in bronchoconstriction in vivo.

If the above hypothesis is true, then we can use the extensive literature on the effects of corticosteroids on various immune functions as a guide to our investigations of the immunologic function of various lipoxygenase products. An example that will be discussed in more detail in the chapter by Dr. Gualde is as follows. Because corticosteroids inhibit the generation of suppressor cells in many in vitro models while NSAIA have no effect in these same models, then there must exist lipoxygenase metabolites that are necessary for suppressor cell generation. Such reasoning led us to find two compounds, LTB_4 and 15-hydroperoxyeicosatetraenoic acid (15-HPETE), that stimulate the generation of suppressor cells in vitro.

I should emphasize that our working hypothesis that corticosteroids work entirely via phospholipase inhibition is not well-accepted (e.g., Reference 9,10) and may very well be incorrect. Nevertheless, it has proven helpful in formulating other, testable hypotheses.

As previously mentioned, it should be clear from Figure 1 that the lipoxygenase metabolites of arachidonic acid are only partially characterized. There may be other lipoxygenases than those listed. In addition, it is probable that each of the hydroperoxyeicosatetraenoic acids formed, which are highly unstable compounds, lead to a cascade of metabolic products analogous to LTA_4, LTB_4, LTC_4, etc. Indeed, Samuelsson et al. have already partially characterized what they term "novel" leukotrienes derived from the 15-lipoxygenase pathway (11), as well as trihydroxy compounds termed "lipoxins." Polyunsaturated fatty acids other than arachidonic acid may also be converted to C-type leukotrienes, but the biological role of these compounds is unknown (12,13).

REFERENCES

1. Gryglewski RJ, Panczenko B, Korbut R, Grodzinska L, Ocetkiewicz A: Corticosteroids inhibit prostaglandin release from perfused mesenteric blood vessels of rabbit and from perfused lungs of sensitized guinea pig. Prostaglandins (10): 343-355, 1975.
2. Kantrowitz F, Robinson DR, McGuire MD, Levine L: Corticosteroids inhibit prostaglandin production by rheumatoid synovia. Nature (258): 737-739, 1975.
3. Floman Y, Zor U: Mechanism of steroid action in inflammation: inhibition of prostaglandin synthesis and release. Prostaglandins (12): 403-413, 1976.
4. Tashjian AH, Voelkel EF, McDonough J, Levine L: Hydrocortisone inhibits prostaglandin production by mouse fibrosarcoma cells. Nature (258): 739-741, 1975.
5. Danon A, Assouline G: Inhibition of prostaglandin biosynthesis by corticosteroids requires RNA and protein synthesis. Nature (173): 552-554, 1978.
6. Flower RJ, Blackwell GJ: Antiinflammatory steroids induce biosynthesis of a phospholipase A_2 inhibitor which prevents prostaglandin generation. Nature (278): 456-459, 1978.
7. Blackwell GJ, Carnuccio R, DiRose M, Glower RJ, Parente L, Perrico P: Macrocortin: a polypeptide causing the antiphospholipase effect of glucocorticoids. Nature (287): 147-149, 1980.

8. Hirata F, Schiffmann E, Venkatasubramanian K, Salomon D, Axelrod J: A phospholipase A_2 inhibitory protein in rabbit neutrophils induced by glucocorticoids. Proc Nat Acad Sci (77): 2533-2536, 1980.
9. Chandrabose KA, Lapetina E, Schmitges C, Siegel M, Cuatrecasas P: Action of corticosteroids in regulation of prostaglandin biosynthesis in cultured fibroblasts. Proc Nat Acad Sci (75): 214-217, 1978.
10. Moore PK, Hoult J: Anti-inflammatory steroids reduce tissue PG synthetase activity and enhance PG breakdown. Nature (288): 269-270, 1980.
11. Jubiz W, Radmark O, Lindgren J, Malsten C, Samuelsson B: Novel leukotrienes: products formed by initial oxygenation of arachidonic acid at C-15. Biochem Biophys Res Comm (99): 976-981, 1981.
12. Hammarström S: Leukotrienes. Ann Rev Biochem (52): 355-377, 1983.
13. Goldman DW, Pickett WC, Goetzl EJ: Human neutrophil chemotactic and degranulating activities of leukotriene B_5 derived from eicosapentaenoic acid. Biochem Biophys Res Comm (117): 282-288, 1983.

Chapter 1

PROSTAGLANDINS, CELLULAR IMMUNITY AND CANCER

JAMES S. GOODWIN and JAN L. CEUPPENS

1. INTRODUCTION

This chapter reviews the literature linking prostaglandins (PGs) to the regulation of the cellular immune response, and includes a discussion of the potential for cyclooxygenase inhibitors used as immuno stimulants in cancer. Most of the work on arachidonic acid metabolites in immunity has been concentrated on the role of PGE in the regulation of cellular and humoral immune responses as well as on monocyte and natural killer (NK) cell function. It is not clear that other cyclooxygenase metabolites--thromboxane, prostacyclin, PGF--play a real role in immune responses. More recently, the effects of lipoxygenase products on immune responses has received increasing attention. This review will focus on the evidence linking PGE to control of cellular immune responses.

The role of PGE in immunoregulation is complex. PGE concentration, state of differentiation of the target cell, and length of PGE-target cell interaction all seem to be important factors whose complete roles have not been delineated. What should not get lost in the midst of this confusion, however, is the solid in vivo and in vitro evidence, reviewed below, that PGE does play a role in immunoregulation. What should also be evident is that the immunomodulatory role of PGE is a fairly minor one, at least in normal organisms. It is clearly not critical for continued functioning, because man and experimental animals do quite well on long term cyclooxygenase inhibitors. What makes the PGE immunomodulatory system especially relevant is two things. First, it is easily inhibited in vivo and in vitro with relatively safe pharmacologic agents, the

J.S. Goodwin (ed.), PROSTAGLANDINS AND IMMUNITY.

non-steroidal anti-inflammatory agents (NSAIA). Second, there exist certain disease states or human conditions associated with decreased cellular immune responses where overactivity of the PGE modulatory system would appear to be at least partially responsible for the immunosuppression. These ideas will be further explored later in this review.

PGE_2 is produced in every tissue examined except mature erythrocytes. The short half life of this compound limits its activity to the site of production. Production in a given tissue is initiated by a stimulus in that tissue, and the PGE_2 then modifies further response to that stimulus. For example, vasopressin stimulates the production of PGE_2 in the distal nephron; PGE_2 in turn makes the collecting duct less sensitive to the action of vasopressin in increasing water permeability (1).

Several pharmacologic agents can affect PG synthesis. Recently, the stimulating effect of nitroglycerin (NTG) on prostacyclin synthesis by human endothelial cells was described, thereby providing a basis for the vasodilating effect of this drug (2). Steroids inhibit the enzyme phospholipase, thereby blocking the release of arachidonic acid, while non-steroidal anti-inflammatory agents such as indomethacin interfere with cyclooxygenase activity (3). Inhibitors of the thromboxane pathway [e.g., imidazole (4), and 9, 11-azoprosta-5, 13-dienoic acid (5)] and of the prostacyclin pathway [e.g., tranylcypromine (6)] have also been synthesized.

It has to be emphasized that "specific" cyclooxygenase inhibitors have actions other than on PG synthesis. Even in submicromolar concentrations, indomethacin is not a specific PG synthetase inhibitor. At 10^{-8}M it inhibits cyclic AMP-dependent protein kinase (7) and at higher concentrations it inhibits phosphodiesterase (8).

2. PGE_2 AS A FEEDBACK INHIBITOR OF CELLULAR IMMUNE FUNCTIONS

That inhibition of immune function by endogenous PGs represents a physiologic feedback mechanism in vivo was first shown by Webb and Osheroff (9), who found that injection of mice with sheep red blood cells led to an 80-fold increase in intrasplenic PG. Prior administration of a PG synthetase inhibitor prevented the PG increase and also resulted in a significantly increased number of plaque-forming spleen cells 3 to 5 d after sensitization. Thus antigen challenge initiated PG production as a negative feedback mechanism.

We examined the effects of PGs on mitogen-stimulated ^{3}H-thymidine incorporation in human peripheral blood mononuclear cells (PBMC) (10). We found that PGE_1 or PGE_2 but not PGA, $PGF_1\alpha$ or $PGF_2\alpha$, inhibited ^{3}H-thymidine incorporation when added in small concentrations (10^{-9} to 10^{-6}M) to concanavalin A (Con A)- or phytohemagglutinin (PHA)-stimulated cultures of PBMC. PGE did not inhibit pokeweed mitogen (PWM) stimulation of PBMC, but did inhibit PWM stimulation of purified T cells. Since PHA and Con A stimulate T cells, while PWM is primarily a B cell mitogen, these data suggest that PGE inhibits T cell, but not B cell mitogenesis. This lack of sensitivity of proliferating B cells to inhibition by PGE depends on the assay employed. B cell colony formation in soft agar is inhibited by nanamolar concentrations of PGE_2 while proliferation of B cells in suspension cultures is insensitive to micromolar concentrations of PGE (11). Actually, this same system-dependent sensitivity to PGE has been shown for T cells, with T colony formation in soft agar inhibited by concentrations as low as 10^{-12}M PGE (12). Whatever the system employed, it would appear that T cell proliferation is more sensitive to inhibition by PGE than is B cell proliferation by several orders of magnitude. PGE_2 is produced in PHA-stimulated cultures of PBMC in amounts that, when added exogenously, causes significant inhibition of mitogen stimulation (10,13). Since PGE_2 is produced in sufficient quantities in PHA cultures to cause an inhibition of ^{3}H-thymidine incorporation in those cultures, one would expect that the addition of PG synthetase inhibitors to PHA cultures would result in increased ^{3}H-thymidine incorporation. This phenomenon is demonstrated in Table 1 at seven different

Table 1. Percentage increase in ^3H-thymidine incorporation caused by indomethacin as a function of dose of mitogen.

PHA concentration	Without indomethacin	With indomethacin	Increase with indomethacin
(μg/ml)	cpm*		%
0.2	411 ± 213	4,764 ± 3,155	1,059 ± 134
0.4	4,823 ± 1,556	16,069 ± 1,724	233 ± 86
1.0	18,164 ± 3,410	35,533 ± 6,281	101 ± 33
2.0	27,768 ± 5,569	47,205 ± 5,591	70 ± 10
4.0	33,079 ± 5,876	56,630 ± 7,378	71 ± 10
8.0	43,428 ± 8,923	60,777 ± 11,753	40 ± 6
20.0	52,111 ± 16,428	54,196 ± 17,197	4 ± 3

*The data are expressed as mean ± SEM of cpm, and of percentage increase in ^3H-thymidine incorporation, in three experiments on different subjects. [Reprinted from (13) with permission of J Clin Invest.]

concentrations of PHA. It is clear that addition of indomethacin enhances ^3H-thymidine incorporation in PHA cultures, and that indomethacin causes a greater percentage increase in ^3H-thymidine incorporation as the dose of PHA is decreased. Similar results were obtained with RO-20-5720, an experimental cyclooxygenase inhibitor which is chemically unrelated to indomethacin (14). One possible explanation for this varying response to PG synthetase inhibitors depending on the concentration of PHA might be that the PBMC are more sensitive to the inhibiting effects of endogenous PGE_2 at lower concentrations of mitogen. This indeed appears to be the case. When several concentrations of PGE_2 are added to cultures containing different amounts of PHA, a family of inhibitory curves is generated, cultures with the lowest concentrations of PHA showing the greatest sensitivity to exogenously added PGE_2. This would appear to be a general rule for all inhibitors: the lower the mitogen dose, the more sensitive the culture is to inhibition (15).

Physiologic concentrations of PGE_2 (10^{-8}M or less) comparable to those found in inflammatory sites (16) have now been shown by several authors to suppress most in vitro manifestations of T lymphocyte functions: mitogen responsiveness (13,17), clonal proliferation (12,18,19) antigenic stimulation (20), E-rosette formation (21,22), lymphokine production [including interleukin 2 (IL2)] (22-26), the generation of cytotoxic cells in mixed lymphocyte culture (27,28), and lymphocyte migration (29,30). Decreased IL2 production contributes to the decreased T cell proliferation caused by PGE_2 (25,31-33), but it is not the only mechanism; the proliferative response of IL2-dependent cells to added IL2 is also inhibited by small concentrations (10^{-9}M) of PGE_2 (24,25,31-33). The cytotoxic activity of non-T lymphocytes, namely NK, antibody-dependent, and monocyte cytotoxic activity, are also inhibited by PGE_2 (34-38). However, it should be mentioned here, as will be further discussed, that under certain experimental conditions PGE_2 can enhance NK activity (39).

The role of arachidonic acid derivatives other than PGE on T cell functions is less clear. Prostacyclin analogues inhibit mitogen stimulation of human lymphocytes (40,41). Some pharmacological products, but not others, that selectively block the synthesis of thromboxane or the lipoxygenase pathways also inhibit mitogenesis (42-44). Thus, it is possible, but far from certain, that thromboxane A_2 (TxA_2) and some lipoxygenase metabolites may promote lymphocyte function. At least two products of the various lipoxygenase pathways, 15-hydroperoxy-eicosatetraenoic acid (15-HPETE) and leukotriene B_4, inhibit T cell functions in vitro, such as mitogen-induced proliferation, E-rosette formation, and lymphokine production (45,46). This will be discussed more fully in the chapter by Dr. Gualde.

3. THE PGE_2-PRODUCING SUPPRESSOR CELL

In human peripheral blood, the cell responsible for PGE_2 production is a monocyte (47,48), while there is evidence in mice that T cells also produce large amounts of PGE (49). Monocytes exposed to mitogens (10,50), endotoxins (51), zymosan (52), interferon (53), antigen-antibody complexes (54), or Fc fragments of IgG (50) increase their PGE_2 production. Immune stimulation thus seems to induce a mechanism tempering the intensity of the response.

An increased activity of the PG-producing suppressor cell has been shown in several chronic inflammatory conditions, including coccidiomytosis (55), Brucella abortus infections in cattle (56), multiple sclerosis (57), rheumatoid arthritis (58-61), experimental cutaneous leishmaniasis (62), nephrotic syndrome (63), tuberculosis (64-66), Q fever (67), Chagas' disease (68), filariasis (69) and sarcoidosis (70). It appears that at least part of the anergy seen in these conditions is due to PG-mediated immunosuppressive activity of macrophages. Muscoplat's group has used in vitro PG blockade as a tool to distinguish cattle previously exposed to Brucella abortus but unresponsive to the antigen, from nonexposed cattle (56). PBMC from previously exposed but anergic cattle, as well as from non-exposed animals, will not respond to Brucella antigen in vitro. After addition of indomethacin to the cultures, PBMC from the previously exposed anergic animals give a positive response to Brucella, while PBMC from the unexposed animals remain unresponsive. This would suggest that PGs are involved in specific immunosuppression against Brucella in the anergic animals. Analogous data have been collected in humans with disseminated Q fever (67) or filariasis (69). It would appear that in patients with disseminated Q fever, an antigen-specific suppressor T cell recognized by the OKT8 monoclonal antibody produces a lymphokine upon exposure to coxiella antigen, and this lymphokine then causes monocytes to increase production of PGE_2. Thus, though the suppression is antigen-specific in elicitation, requiring the specific coxiella antigen, the subsequent suppression is antigen-nonspecific, being mediated by PGE_2 (67).

The depressed PHA response of PBMC from patients with disseminated coccidiomycosis can be reversed with indomethacin (55).

It was not possible, however, to reverse the specific anergy to the infecting agent. Thus PBMC from subjects with disseminated coccidiomycosis did not respond to coccidioidin in vitro even with indomethacin in the cultures. This is clearly different from the case with brucellosis and coxiella described above.

PG-mediated suppression has also been studied in the depressed cellular immunity associated with sarcoidosis (70). The depressed PHA response of patients with sarcoidosis could be largely reversed by removing the glass-adherent cells but not by inhibition of PG synthesis. The depressed mitogen response of patients with rheumatoid arthritis would also appear to be secondary to suppressor monocytes that are working by other mechanisms in addition to increased PGE production (58-61). These findings support the contention of Rice et al. (71) and others (72,73) that there are at least two monocyte suppressor mechanisms in human PBMC, only one of which is dependent on PG synthesis. The other suppressor mechanism in monocytes would appear to involve hydrogen peroxide production (74).

Plasma of patients with tuberculosis contains a factor (probably a mycobacterial wall antigen, alone or bound in immune complexes) that inhibits the proliferation of normal lymphocytes through enhancement of PG synthesis (64). Increased PG production by adherent cells is also observed during a graft versus host (GVH) response and is responsible in part for GVH-induced immunosuppression (75). Efferent lymph from nodes of sheep challenged with antigen was found to suppress the in vitro transformation of peripheral blood lymphocytes to a variety of antigens, and the suppressor factor was shown to be PGE_2 (76).

It is interesting to note that in some experimental animal models the depressed immune response was reversed with in vivo indomethacin administration but not with addition of indomethacin directly to cultures of lymphocytes from these animals (63). Thus some PG-mediated suppression can be reversed in vivo but not in vitro.

Administration of anti-thymocyte antisera to monkeys induces circulating PGE-producing suppressor cells (77), raising the possibility that the increase in activity of these cells seen in various rheumatic diseases may be secondary to endogenous production of these autoantibodies.

4. CHANGES IN SENSITIVITY OF LYMPHOCYTES TO PGE_2

Changes in the sensitivity of lymphocytes to PGE_2 have been observed in several instances.

a) Lymphocytes from normal individuals with the HLA-B12 haplotype have a decreased sensitivity to PGs and histamine, and this could play a role in propensity for autoimmune disorders in these subjects (45,78).

b) Lymphocytes from patients with multiple sclerosis exhibit a defective response to PGE_2 in one assay system (79) but not in another (80). Further evidence for an actual role for PGE in this disease is provided by a study from Zurier's laboratory showing that lymphocytes from patients with multiple sclerosis have an increased adherence to measles-infected cells which can be reversed in vitro or in vivo by the administration of PG synthetase inhibitors (57,81).

c) Page and co-workers have reported that lymphocytes from patients with juvenile periodontitis are less sensitive to inhibition by PGE_2 (10^{-5}M) than are cells from patients with adult periodontitis or normal controls (82). They postulate that a defect in the response of lymphocytes to PGE_2 allows for the exuberant immune reactivity seen in subjects with juvenile periodontitis.

d) Lymphocytes from healthy subjects over age 70 are much more sensitive to inhibition by exogenous PGE_2 than are PBMC from young adults (83-87). The amount of PGE_2 required to cause 50% inhibition of the PHA response of healthy subjects over age 70 is approximately 10^{-8}M. This is more than two orders of magnitude lower than the amount required for 50% inhibition in young adults ($> 3 \times 10^{-6}$M). This increased sensitivity to PGE would appear to contribute to some of the disturbances in cellular and humoral immune function found in healthy old people (83,86,87).

e) One of the fascinating questions confronting immunologists is how the fetus with its complement of paternal antigens escapes immunologic rejection by the mother (88). Several groups of investigators have demonstrated suppressor cells in the spleens of fetal mice or in human cord blood that strongly inhibit maternal T cell functions such as proliferation (88-90). More recently, Olding and his colleagues have reported that suppression of maternal lymphocyte mitogenesis by newborn cells can be reversed with indomethacin (91). While newborn lymphocytes suppress maternal lymphocyte mitogen responses across a semi-permeable membrane, lymphocytes from one newborn do not suppress the mitogen responses of lymphocytes from another newborn (91). In other words, PG-mediated suppression by newborn lymphocytes selectively affects maternal lymphocytes and not newborn lymphocytes. It would appear that lymphocytes from newborns are insensitive to inhibition by PGE (92 and L.B. Olding et al., submitted for publication), while maternal lymphocytes may have increased sensitivity to PGE_2 (92), though this latter finding is disputed (93).

f) An increased sensitivity to PGE_2 was observed after surgery and in women in labor (94). Thus it would appear that physical stress causes lymphocytes to become more sensitive to PGE_2, and the increased sensitivity to inhibition by this endogenous immunomodulator is responsible in part for the depressed cellular immune function following physical stress. In mice, the depressed cellular immune reactivity of splenocytes after surgical trauma can be reversed with indomethacin (95); in humans after surgery the reversal by indomethacin in vitro of depressed lymphocyte PHA responses is only partial (94).

g) Lymphocytes from patients with rheumatoid arthritis also are more sensitive than normal to inhibition by exogenous PGE_2 (58,96). This finding may be relevant to the selective loss of normal immunoregulation in the joints of patients with rheumatoid arthritis (97,98).

h) Kelly et al. (99) examined inhibition of production of leukocyte migration inhibitory factor (LIF) in PHA-stimulated cultures by PGE_2 and found that lymphocytes from patients with scleroderma were insensitive to inhibition by PGE_2. These investigators concluded that this lack of sensitivity to a normal "turn off" signal may be responsible for lymphokine-stimulated accumulation of connective tissue in this disease.

Because similar defects in sensitivity to PGE are seen in such disparate conditions as multiple sclerosis, scleroderma and juvenile periodontitis (see above), it is difficult to imagine that the loss of sensitivity to PGE is the actual cause of the condition. At least as likely is the possibility that the chronic inflammatory process leads somehow to a loss of PGE sensitivity in lymphocytes. It is interesting in this regard to note that in some in vitro systems, maintenance of cellular sensitivity to PGE is an active process modulated by lymphokines (100).

5. EFFECT OF PG SYNTHETASE INHIBITORS ON CELLULAR IMMUNE FUNCTIONS IN VIVO.

Cyclooxygenase inhibitors in vivo stimulate cellular immune responses in humans and experimental animals (101-107). Muscoplat et al. studied the effect of indomethacin administration on delayed hypersensitivity skin responses in guinea pigs previously sensitized to mycobacterium bovis (102). Oral administration of indomethacin simultaneous with intradermal injection of Mycobacterium bovis antigen resulted in a more than two-fold increase in skin thickness compared to the guinea pigs not given indomethacin. Delayed skin test responses to other antigens were also shown to be enhanced by indomethacin in guinea pigs (103).

Inhibition of endogenous PG biosynthesis by indomethacin shortened allograft survival in mice, and this effect was completely abrogated by concurrent injections of a PGE_2 analogue (104). Another in vivo correlate of the immunosuppressive activity of PGE_2 is that local injection of PGE_2 can cause reactivation of herpes simplex infection in the mouse ear (105). Natural killer cell activity is also enhanced in vivo by PG synthesis inhibitors. Brunda et al. have shown that in vivo administration of indomethacin or aspirin resulted in a marked restoration of NK activity in tumor-bearing animals (44). Tracey and Adkinson showed that the BCG augmentation of NK activity could be further potentiated by indomethacin in vivo (and in vitro) (106). On the other hand, aspirin ingestion by normal volunteers within 48 h of blood drawing results in a decrease in NK activity in certain assay systems (108).

The effect of indomethacin administration in man on delayed hypersensitivity skin testing has also been studied (101,107). Indomethacin administration (100 mg/d) for 5 d did not influence the amount of induration caused by a battery of three common antigens in 10 normal subjects (107). As shown in Figure 1, when indomethacin was administered to subjects with depressed cellular immunity there was an enhancement of delayed hypersensitivity (101). Two previously anergic patients with common variable immunodeficiency became reactive to skin tests while on indomethacin (100 mg/d) and became anergic again after the medication was stopped. The in vitro response of the patients' lymphocytes to PHA also rose while they were taking indomethacin. Enhancement of mitogen responses in patients with rheumatoid arthritis who are put on NSAIA has been found in two studies (97,109) but not in another (110).

In summary, several in vivo and ex vivo studies confirm the in vitro experiments showing that PGE acts as a feedback inhibitor of cellular immune responses and that these responses can be enhanced in vivo as well as in vitro by administration of cyclooxygenase inhibitors.

6. CELLULAR ACTIVATION BY PGE_2

Until now we have discussed immunosuppressive activities of PGE_2 on immunocyte function. It is clear, however, that under certain experimental conditions PGE_2 can deliver activating signals. For example, PGE induces immature thymocytes to differentiate into mature T cells (111). Indeed, it would appear that thymic hormones act via stimulation of PGE synthesis (112)

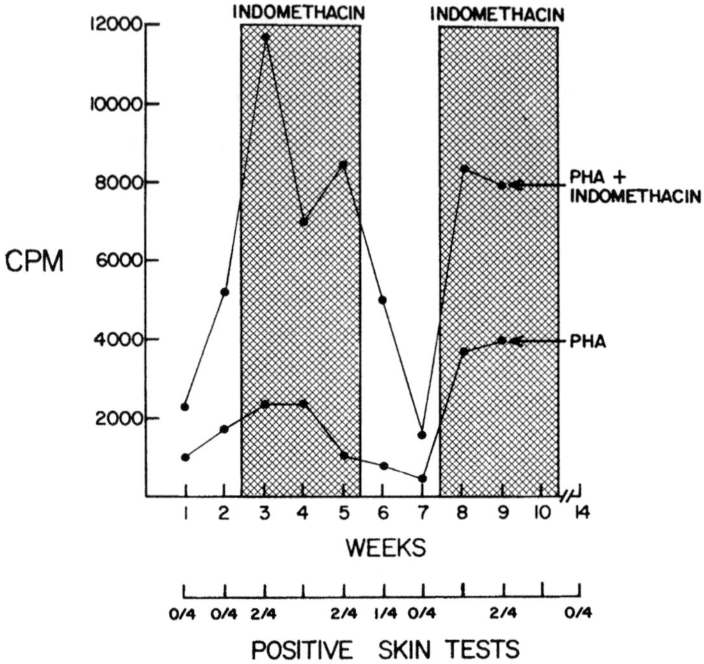

FIGURE 1. Effect of indomethacin administration on delayed hypersensitivity skin testing and mitogen-induced T cell proliferation in a patient with adult combined immunodeficiency. The shaded area represents the period of indomethacin administration (100 mg/d in divided doses). The top part of the figure plots the PHA response, with or without indomethacin added in vitro. Indomethacin administration in vivo was associated with a reversible increase in PHA response and in delayed hypersensitivity skin testing. The positive skin tests were > 10 mm induration, while the negative tests showed no induration. [Reproduced from (101) with permission of J Clin Lab Immunol.]

and that NSAIA block the action of thymic hormone in vivo (113). Analogous data have been obtained with B cell differentiation, with PGE stimulating the appearance of Fc receptors on immature B cell lines (114). In multiple sclerosis patients, an increased production of PGE_2 by the monocytes causes increased adherence of the lymphocytes to measles-infected cells (81) and an increased number of active E-rosette-forming lymphocytes (115).

PGE also causes activation of suppressor cells in some assay systems, as will be discussed by Dr. Fischer and his colleagues.

Stobo and associates have shown that PGE_2 can increase the mitogenic reactivity of preincubated low density T cells (116), while it decreases the reactivity of medium and high density T cells. These investigators concluded that PGE_2 should be considered a regulator rather than a universal suppressor for T cell reactivity. More recently, we have shown that the suppressor-cytotoxic subset of T cells, as defined by the monoclonal antibody OKT8, has an increased mitogen-induced proliferation with exposure to PGE if the cells are first preincubated (117).

Dual effects (inhibition or activation) of PGE have been observed on B cells, NK cells and macrophages. A short exposure of PBMC to PGE_2 followed by a 24-h incubation increases NK activity, while PGE_2 added during effector-target cell interaction inhibited NK activity (118). PGE_2 can both enhance and block NK activation by interferon (39). Interferon-induced and lipopolysaccharide (LPS)-induced tumoricidal activity of monocytes are inhibited by high doses of PGE_2 (100,119), but indomethacin inhibits and PGE_2 restores endotoxin-induced tumoricidal activity of macrophages (72). Other authors have shown that PGE reduces the cytotoxic effect of BCG-activated macrophages but enhances the growth-inhibitory capacity of normal macrophages (120). The authors suggested that PGE may play a role in regulating macrophage function based on the level of activation of the macrophage. Phagocytosis by macrophages has been shown to be enhanced by PGE_2 by some investigators and inhibited by others (121,122). Small concentrations of PGE_2 (10^{-9}M) cause suppression of macrophage spreading and adherence, while larger concentrations (10^{-7} and 10^{-6}M) cause enhanced migration (122). Endotoxins and lymphokines induce collagenase production by macrophages, and this production is dependent on a rise in cyclic AMP induced by PGE_2 (123). Collagenase production is blocked by indomethacin and restored by exogenous PGE_2.

It should be clear from these data that PGE cannot be considered as a universal cell inhibitor and that its physiologic role is very complex. As mentioned above, the PGE concentration, the activation and differentiation status of the target cell, and the length of PGE-target cell interaction all seem to be important factors whose complete roles have not been fully delineated.

7. MECHANISM OF ACTION OF PGE_2 AT THE CELLULAR LEVEL

Most attention has been focused on the effect of PGE_2 on intracellular cyclic AMP. PGE_2 activates adenylate cyclase with a subsequent rise in cyclic AMP (124). Cyclic AMP itself is an inhibitor of lymphocyte activation (124,125). We and others have addressed the possibility that cyclic AMP is a second messenger for the action of PGE_2 in several studies. We have demonstrated the presence of receptors for PGE_1 and PGE_2 on the lymphocyte surface, while there were no binding sites for PGA, $PGF_1\alpha$ or $PGF_2\alpha$ (126). The dissociation constant (Kd) for PGE_2 binding was 2×10^{-9}M and the B max was 200 binding sites per cell, assuming uniform distribution. These binding sites for PGE_2 are lost during overnight incubation, which parallels the loss of the inhibitory effect of PGE_2 on the mitogenic stimulation of preincubated lymphocytes (3,19,127). PGE, but not PGF, caused increases in intracellular cyclic AMP in lymphocytes, and this effect was also lost with preincubation (128). Thus the functional effects (inhibition of mitogenesis), the cell surface receptors, and the cyclic AMP response share a specificity for PGE over PGF, and all are lost with preincubation. Webb et al. demonstrated by cyclic AMP extraction and by direct fluorescence visualization an increase in intracellular cyclic AMP in spleen cells after antigenic challenge with sheep red blood cells, which is dependent on a concomitant increase in PG levels (9,129). T cells bearing a receptor for the Fc portion of IgG (Tγ cells) had a 27-fold rise in cyclic AMP after exposure to PGE_2 whereas the remaining T cells had a four-fold increase (130). Tγ cells have been shown by Moretta et al. to be suppressive for PWM-driven B cell differentiation into plasma cells (131). Thus, suppressor T cells have a high density of PGE_2 receptors on their membranes relative to helper cells.

It should be noted that the link between PGE effects and cyclic AMP is not entirely established, and the possibility still exists that many of the effects of PGE on immune function are mediated in ways independent of adenylate cyclase stimulation.

8. PROSTAGLANDINS AND TUMOR GROWTH

Tumors, just as other antigenic stimuli, lead to increased activity of the PG-producing suppressor cell. Pelus and Bockman (132) showed that macrophages from tumor-bearing mice produced significantly more PGE than cells from normal littermates. The existence of indomethacin-sensitive adherent suppressor cells has also been shown by Glasser in tumor-bearing mice (133). Spleen cells of tumor-bearing mice inhibited the in vitro generation of secondary cytotoxic reactivity of spleen cells of tumor-free mice, sensitized in vitro with SV-40-induced tumor cells. The suppressor cells were shown to be macrophages, and indomethacin eliminated the suppressive activity.

Studies of patients with various types of cancer demonstrated overactivity of the PG-producing suppressor cell. We have investigated the role of the PG-producing suppressor cell in the hyporesponsiveness to PHA of PBMC from patients with Hodgkin's disease (134). Six patients with untreated Hodgkin's disease, nodular sclerosing type, were studied. The mean response of the Hodgkin's disease lymphocytes was 48% of the mean control response. This increased to 94% of normal with addition of indomethacin. Thus indomethacin almost totally reversed the depressed PHA response in Hodgkin's disease lymphocytes. The suppression of the PHA response in the patients with Hodgkin's disease was also reversed by removal of glass-adherent cells prior to culture. This was expected, since the PG-producing suppressor cells are glass-adherent (10).

PGE_2 production was then measured in mitogen cultures of PBMC from three patients with Hodgkin's disease and three age and sex-matched controls. The mean PGE_2 production of the Hodgkin's disease PBMC was 20,600 ± 7620 pg/ml (6×10^{-8}M) in 48 h versus 6368 ± 2944 pg/ml (1.6×10^{-8}M) for the controls (mean ± SD, $P < 0.02$). The amount of PGE_2 produced in the cultures of Hodgkin's disease lymphocytes caused 65% inhibition when added exogenously to Hodgkin's disease glass-nonadherent cells, while the amount of PGE_2 produced by the controls caused 35% inhibition when added to normal glass-nonadherent cells. Other studies have confirmed the increased activity of the PG-producing suppressor cell in Hodgkin's disease (135-138), but these studies reported only a partial reversal of depressed T cell responses in vitro with addition of indomethacin.

In other human cancers, the evidence that overactivity of the normal PGE feedback inhibition is a major contribution to T cell dysfunction is less clear. In ten anergic patients with a variety of metastatic solid tumors, the enhancement of mitogen responses with indomethacin was only slightly greater than control (139). Vosixa and Thies, in a study of 24 cancer patients, found an increased activity of the PG-producing suppressor cell in 6 of 24 patients (140). Similar reports have been published from other laboratories (141-143). However, in all of these studies the patients' responses remained quite depressed after indomethacin.

Apart from activation of the PG-producing suppressor cell, tumor cells themselves can produce immunodepressing PGE. The first data about PGE_2 production by tumors came from investigators interested in the mechanism of hypercalcemia associated with cancer not metastatic to bone. PGE_2 is a potent stimulator of bone resorption in vitro (144). Enhanced PGE production by naturally occurring or experimentally induced cancers has now been documented in several studies (144-151). Droller and coworkers, using a carcinogen-induced bladder tumor in Fisher rats, showed that direct contact between functionally active lymphocytes and tumor cells is necessary for increased tumor cell protaglandin production to occur (152).

If increased PG production by the tumor and by host macrophages is important in inhibiting the immune response of the host--especially in the immediate environment of the tumor--and in allowing the tumor to escape immunologic rejection, then one would expect that administration of PG synthesis inhibitors in vivo to experimental tumor-bearing animals or cancer patients would result in: 1) an improvement in immune function, and 2) retardation of tumor growth.

That this can occur in vivo was first shown by Plescia and coworkers (153,154). Administration of PG synthesis inhibitors to tumor-bearing mice resulted in restoration of the antibody response to sheep erythrocytes and in slowing of tumor growth. Several other laboratories have achieved similar results. Brunda et al. demonstrated that splenocytes from mice with Moloney virus-induced sarcomas had severely suppressed NK activity, and that this NK activity could be restored to normal by administration of aspirin or indomethacin in vivo (35). Hial et al. administered aspirin or indomethacin to mice that had received a mast cell ascites tumor or Lewis lung carcinoma (155). Both drugs in normal therapeutic doses caused a substantial slowing of the growth of both tumors. At higher indomethacin doses (5 mg/kg/d) there was elimination of the tumors in 50% of the cases, but there were also signs of gastric toxicity and weight loss in the mice. In these studies, as in the ones by Plescia, the PG synthetase inhibitors were started simultaneously with tumor inoculation. When there was a delay between tumor inoculation and drug administration, the anti-tumor effects were less pronounced. Lynch et al. reported that indomethacin and aspirin inhibited the growth of a methylcholanthrene-induced fibrosarcoma in mice (156). The drugs were not started until 7 d after tumor inoculation, when the tumor was already palpable. In approximately 20% of the indomethacin-treated mice, the tumor completely regressed and did not reappear after cessation of the drug. Strausser and colleagues have reported that indomethacin will delay the onset and slow the growth of Moloney sarcoma virus-induced tumors in mice (157,158). If the drug is started at the same time as virus injection, no tumors develop. Bennett et al. reported that treatment with flurbiprofen (an inhibitor of PG synthesis) started before injection of mammary cancer cells reduced tumor growth and lengthened the survival time of mice (159). Indomethacin started 14 d after injection of a carcinogen reduced significantly the appearance of intestinal tumor in a study by Pollard and Luckert (160). There are also now at least two reports of regression of human cancers after ingestion of a NSAIA (161,162). It is not unrealistic to expect that cyclooxygenase inhibitors may prove a useful adjuvant in the treatment of certain human cancers in the future. Given the experience with the B16 melanoma described below, however, it may very well be that some human cancers will get worse on these drugs. We feel that the data in experimental animals is sufficiently compelling to justify careful trials in humans.

In most of these studies it is not clear that the inhibition of tumor growth is indeed induced by an effect on the immune system. Lynch et al., while confirming that the administration of PG synthetase inhibition does slow the growth of or eliminate many experimental tumors, dispute the claim that these drugs work via stimulation of the host's immune system (156). They showed that mice that had completely eliminated their tumors with indomethacin treatment were not immune to rechallenge with the same tumor. Augmentation of the immune response in tumor-bearing mice by indomethacin did not correlate with the anti-tumor effects of the drug. The data are, however, still consistent with the possibility that PG synthetase inhibition works via augmentation of NK activity and macrophage cytotoxicity, neither of which demonstrate immunologic memory.

There are indications that inhibition of PG synthesis can inhibit tumor metastasis by mechanisms not related to the immune system. PGs may have a role in the establishment of bone metastases (163,164). PGE is indeed a powerful stimulus for bone resorption (144) and is necessary for the production of osteoclast activating factor by leukocytes (165).

Finally, we should consider the effect of PGs and of PG synthetase inhibitors on carcinogenesis and on the tumor cells themselves. This effect can be different, according to the tumor type studied. The formation of squamous cell carcinoma was shown to be markedly enhanced by concomitant PGE_2 and $PGF_2\alpha$ administration to mice treated with 3-methylcholanthrene for two months (166). Carcinogens such as TPA (a phorbolester) or polycyclic aromatic hydrocarbons increase PGE production of the target cells (167-169). A positive correlation was found between carcinogenicity and stimulation of PG production. Cycloheximide inhibited the TPA-induced morphological changes and PG synthesis (168). It is therefore possible that PGs are involved in the actions of these tumor promotors. Buick et al. studied the clonigenic capacity of tumor cells obtained from malignant effusions from 31 patients with epithelial tumors (170). They found that host macrophages stimulated the growth of these cells in vitro and that PG synthetase inhibitors eliminated this stimulation. There are also indications that breast cancers with high PGE production are more locally invasive and have a higher tendency for metastatic spread (149).

Not all the evidence, however, points to a beneficial effect of PG synthetase inhibitors to inhibit tumor growth. Some tumor cell lines are inhibited by PGE, while cyclooxygenase inhibitors stimulate their growth (171). Daily injection of a PGE analogue into the site of a B16 melanoma tumor cell inoculation slowed the growth of these tumors by about 60% (171). The B16 melanoma studied is unusual in that its main arachidonic acid metabolite is PGD_2 (172). This same cell line was used in a study showing that PGE_2 administration can improve immune response and survival of tumor-bearing animals (173). Addition of indomethacin to cytotoxic drug regimens resulted in either no change or a decrease in the effectiveness of the chemotherapy against B16 melanoma (174). In another study using the B16 melanoma cell line, Stringfellow and Fitzpatrick showed that PGD_2 production by these tumor cells was inversely correlated with their metastatic potential (172). Exposure of the melanoma cells to indomethacin prior to inoculation resulted in a substantial increase in the rate of pulmonary metastases. PGE_2 added to cultures of erythroleukemia cells in the presence of the inducer DMSO produced 73% inhibition of cell growth (175). The effect of PGs on tumor cell growth can also be dose-dependent. Karmali et al. showed that the proliferation of Raji cells (a cell line derived from a Burkitt lymphoma) is enhanced by PGE_2 in a concentration of 10^{-12} to 10^{-11}M, while doses above 10^{-9}M inhibit cell growth (176).

Disappointing results of clinical trials with nonspecific immune stimulation in cancer patients become more understandable in the light of recent work showing that C. parvum and BCG, in addition to nonspecifically enhancing humoral and cellular immune responses, also induce the generation of suppressor cells in the host animals (177-181). The BCG-induced splenic suppressor cell in mice is adherent, phagocytic and lacks the Thy-1 antigen (178). This macrophage-like cell inhibits NK cell activity, the generation of cytotoxic T cells, mitogen- or alloantigen-induced T cell proliferation and the plaque-forming response to antigens (177-181). A possible mechanism for such macrophage-like suppressor cells is via production of PGs. There are now some data suggesting that PGs may indeed be important in the function of these cells. First, both C. parvum and BCG induce macrophages to increase their PG production more than 50-fold (182,183). Second, BCG causes macrophages to produce factors that stimulate or inhibit NK activity (106). It remains to be seen whether in vivo indomethacin will prevent the late development of splenic suppressor cells and the concomitant late decrease in NK activity, T cell cytotoxicity and humoral immune responses after BCG treatment.

This whole question was given more relevance by the finding that in vivo indomethacin substantially increased the anti-tumor activities of C. parvum and BCG (106,184). In one report, the injection of 10^9 killed C. parvum organisms into fibrosarcoma tumors at 10 d and then again at 17 d after grafting resulted in elimination of the tumor by day 50 (184). However, if the C. parvum injections were given at days 17 and 24, when the tumor was substantially larger, there was no effect on subsequent tumor growth. The addition of indomethacin to this latter regimen resulted in elimination of the tumor in 50% of the cases. Similar findings were reported for BCG. When the C. parvum was given by intraperitoneal injection rather than intratumor, no effect on tumor growth was noted unless indomethacin was also administered, in which case the tumor regressed in 50% of the mice.

Analogous results have been reported with another potential immunoadjuvant, interferon (185,186). The combination of interferon inducers plus indomethacin in vivo caused greater regression of bladder tumors in mice than did either agent alone (186).

9. CONCLUSION

Four years ago, when we reviewed the literature on PGs and immune function, the task was considerably simpler and the story was cleaner (187). The story has become more complex but also more interesting. The possibility that nonsteroidal drugs may play a useful role in the treatment of some human malignancies is as attractive and as unproven as ever. [This chapter is largely based on a review published in The Journal of Clinical Immunology (188), and those parts are reproduced with permission.]

REFERENCES

1. Lum GM, Aisenbrey GA, Dunn RW, Berl RW, Schrier RW, McDonald KM: In vivo effect of indomethacin to potentiate the renal medullary cyclic AMP response to vasopressin. J Clin Invest (59): 8-12, 1977.
2. Levin RI, Jaffe EA, Weksler BB, Tack-Goldman KT: Nitroglycerin stimulates synthesis of prostacyclin by cultured human endothelial cells. J Clin Invest (67): 762-770, 1981.
3. Vane JR: Inhibition of prostaglandin synthesis as a mechanism of action for aspirin-like drugs. Nature New Biol 231-238, 1971.

4. Needleman P, Raz A, Ferrendelli JA, Minkes M: Application of imidazole as a selective inhibitor thromboxane synthetase in human platelets. Proc Natl Acad Sci (74): 1716-1724, 1977.
5. Gorman RR, Bundy GL, Peterson DC, Sun FF, Miller OV, Fitzpatrick FA: Inhibition of human platelet thromboxane synthetase by 9,11-azoprosta-5,13-dienoic acid. Proc Natl Acad Sci (74): 4007-4013, 1977.
6. Gryglewski RJ, Bunting S, Moncada S, Flower RJ, Vane JR: Arterial walls are protected against deposition of platelet thrombic by a substance (prostaglandin x) which they make from prostaglandin endoperoxides. Prostaglandins (12): 685-691, 1976.
7. Kantor HS, Hampton M: Indomethacin in submicromolar concentrations inhibits cyclic AMP-dependent protein kinase. Nature (London) (276): 841-844, 1978.
8. Ciosek CP, Ortel RW, Thanassi NM, Newcombe DS: Inhibition of phosphodiesterase by non-steroidal anti-inflammatory drugs. Nature (London) (251): 148-150, 1974.
9. Webb DR, Osheroff PL: Antigen stimulation of prostaglandin synthesis and control of immune responses. Proc Natl Acad Sci USA (73): 1300-1309, 1976.
10. Goodwin JS, Bankhurst AD, Messner RP: Suppression of human T-cell mitogenesis by prostaglandin; existence of a prostaglandin-producing suppressor cell. J Exp Med (146): 1719-1734, 1977.
11. Whisler RL, Newhouse VG: Inhibition of human B lymphocyte colony responses by endogenous synthesized hydrogen peroxide and prostaglandins. Cell Immunol (69): 34-45, 1982.
12. Eckles DD, Gershwin ME: Pharmacologic and biochemical production of human T-lymphocyte colony formation: hormonal influences. Immunopharmacology (3): 259-274, 1981.
13. Goodwin JS, Messner RP, Peake GT: Prostaglandin suppression of mitogen-stimulated lymphocytes in vitro. J Clin Invest (62): 753-760, 1978.
14. Gaut ZN, Baruth H, Randall LO, Ashley C, Paulsrud JR: Stereoisomeric relationships among anti-inflammatory activity, inhibition of platelet aggregation, and inhibition of prostaglandin synthetase. Prostaglandins (10): 59-65, 1975.
15. Goodwin JS, Messner RP, Williams RC Jr: Inhibitors of T-cell mitogenesis: effect of mitogen dose. Cell Immunol (45): 303-309, 1979.
16. Robinson DR, Levine L: Prostaglandin concentrations in synovial fluid in rheumatic diseases: action of indomethacin and aspirin. In: Robinson HJ, Vane JR (eds) Prostaglandin synthetase inhibitors--their effects on physiological functions and pathological states (symposium). Raven Press, New York, 1974, pp 223-228.
17. Novagrodsky A, Rubin AL, Stenzel KH: Selective suppression by adherent cells, prostaglandin, and cyclic AMP analogues of blastogenesis induced by different mitogens. J Immunol (122): 1-8, 1979.

18. Bockman RS: PGE inhibition of T-lymphocyte colony formation. J Clin Invest (64): 812-821, 1979.
19. Gorski A, Gaciong, Dupont B: Enhanced colonability of human T lymphocytes caused by their culturing in vitro. Immunology (44): 617-622, 1982.
20. Muscoplat CC, Klausner DJ, Brunner CJ, Sloane, ED, Johnson DW: Regulation of mitogen- and antigen-stimulated lymphocyte blastogenesis by prostaglandins. Infect Immun (26): 311-316, 1979.
21. Erten U, Emre T, Cavdar AO, Turker RK: An in vitro study on the effect of prostaglandin E_2 and $F_{2\alpha}$ on E-rosette forming activity on normal lymphocytes. Prostaglandins Med (5): 255-261, 1980.
22. Venza-Teti D, Misefari A, Sofo, V, Fimiani V, La Via ML: Interaction between prostaglandins and human T lymphocytes: effect of PGE_2 on E-receptor expression. Immunopharmacology (2): 165-171, 1980.
23. Gordon D, Bray M, Morley J: Control of lymphokine secretion by prostaglandins. Nature (262): 401-407, 1976.
24. Baker PE, Fahey JV, Munck A: Prostaglandin inhibition of T-cell proliferation is mediated at two levels. Cell Immunol (61): 52-57, 1981.
25. Rappaport RS, Dodge GR: Prostaglandin E inhibits the production of human interleukin 2. J Exp Med (155): 943-948, 1982.
26. Soppi E, Eskola J, Ruuskanen O: Effects of indomethacin on lymphocyte proliferation, suppressor cell function, and leukocyte migration inhibitory factor (LMIF) production. Immunopharmacology (4): 2365-2372, 1982.
27. Darrow TL, Tomar RH: Prostaglandin-mediated regulation of the mixed lymphocyte culture and generation of cytotoxic cells. Cell Immunol (65): 172-178, 1980.
28. Leung KH, Mihich E: Prostaglandin modulation of development of cell-mediated immunity in culture. Nature (288): 597-603, 1980.
29. Van Epps D: Suppression of human lymphocyte migration by PGE_2. Inflammation (5): 81-87, 1981.
30. Hopkins J, McConnell I, Pearson JD: Lymphocyte traffic through antigen-stimulated lymph nodes. Immunology (42): 225-231, 1981.
31. Tilden AB, Blach CM: A comparison of PGE_2 effects on human suppressor cell function and on interleukin 2 function. J Immunol (129): 2469-2473, 1982.
32. Chouaib S, Fradelizi D: The mechanism of inhibition of interleukin 2 production. J Immunol (129): 2463-2468, 1982.
33. Wolf M, Droege W: Inhibition of cytotoxic responses by prostaglandin E_2 in the presence of interleukin 2. Cell Immunol (72): 286-293, 1982.
34. Schultz RM, Stoychkov JN, Pavlidis N, Chirigos MA, Olkowski ZL: Role of E-type prostaglandin in the regulation of interferon-treated macrophage cytotoxic activity. J Reticuloendothel Soc (26): 93-100, 1979.

35. Brunda MJ, Herberman RB, Holden HT: Inhibition of murine natural killer cell activity by prostaglandins. J Immunol (124): 2682-2688, 1980.
36. Garovoy MR, Strom RB, Kaliner M, Carpenter CB: Antibody-dependent lymphocyte mediated cytotoxicity mechanism and modulation by cyclic nucleotides. Cell Immunol (20): 197-205, 1975.
37. Trofatter KF Jr, Daniels CA: Interaction of human cells with prostaglandins and cyclic AMP modulators. I. Effects on complement-mediated lysis and antibody-dependent cell-mediated cytolysis of herpes simplex virus-infected human fibroblasts. J Immunol (122): 1363-1370, 1979.
38. Droller MJ, Schneider MU, Perlmann P: A possible role of prostaglandins in the inhibition of natural and antibody-dependent cell-mediated cytotoxicity against tumor cells. Cell Immunol (39): 165-172, 1978.
39. Targan S: The dual interaction of prostaglandin E_2 (PGE_2) and interferon (IFN) on NK lytic activation: enhanced capacity of effector-target lytic interactions (recycling) and blockage of pre-NK cell recruitment. J Immunol (127): 1424-1430, 1981.
40. Kingston A, Kay JE, Ivanyi J: The effect of prostaglandin E_2 and I_2-analogues on mitogen induced lymphocyte stimulation. Int J Immunopharmacol (2): 243-250, 1980.
41. Gordon D, Henderson DC, Westwick J: Effects of prostaglandins E_2 and I_2 on human lymphocyte transformation in the presence and absence of inhibitors of prostaglandin biosynthesis. Br J Pharmacol (67): 17-20, 1979.
42. Kelly JP, Johnson MC, Parker CW: Effect of inhibitors of arachidonic acid metabolism on mitogenesis in human lymphocytes: possible role of thromboxanes and products of the lipoxygenase pathway. J Immunol (122): 1563-1559, 1979.
43. Leung K, Mihich E: Modulation of cell-mediated immunity of prostaglandin synthesis. Int J Immunopharmacol (2): 244-249, 1980.
44. Gordon D, Novri A, Thomas R: Selective inhibition of thromboxane biosynthesis in human blood mononuclear cells and the effects on mitogen-stimulated lymphocyte proliferation. Immunology (42): 472-478, 1981.
45. Gualde N, Rabinovitch H, Fredon M, Rigaud M: Effects of 15-hydroperoxyeicosatetraenoic acid on human lymphocyte sheep erythrocyte rosette formation and response to concanavalin A associated with HLA system. Eur J Immunol (12): 773-777, 1982.
46. Goetzl E, Payan DG, Goetzl EJ: Specific suppression of human T lymphocyte function by leukotriene B4. J Immunol (131): 551-553, 1983.
47. Kennedy MS, Stobo JD, Goldyne ME: In vitro synthesis of prostaglandins and related lipids by populations of human peripheral blood mononuclear cells. Prostaglandins (20): 135-141, 1980.

48. Kurland JI, Bockman R: Prostaglandin E production by human blood monocytes and mouse peritoneal macrophages. J Exp Med (147): 952-960, 1978.
49. Webb DR, Nowowiejski I: Mitogen-induced changes in lymphocyte prostaglandin levels: a signal for the induction of suppressor cell activity. Cell Immunol (41): 72-78, 1978.
50. Passwell JH, Dayer JM, Merler E: Increased prostaglandin production by human monocytes after membrane receptor activation. J Immunol (123): 115-121, 1979.
51. Humes JL, Bonney RJ, Pelus L, Dahlgren ME, Sadowski SJ, Kuehl FA Jr, Davies P: Macrophages synthesise and release prostaglandins in response to inflammatory stimuli. Nature (269): 149-150, 1977.
52. Ellner JJ, Spagnvolo PJ: Suppression of antigen and mitogen induced human T lymphocyte DNA synthesis by bacterial lipopolysaccharide; mediation by monocyte activation and production of prostaglandins. J Immunol (123): 2689-2695, 1979.
53. Fuse A, Mahmud I, Kuwata T: Mechanism of stimulation by interferon of prostaglandin synthesis in human cell lines. Cancer Res (42): 3209-3214, 1982.
54. Bonney RJ, Naruns PP, Davies P, Humes JL: Antigen-antibody complexes stimulate the synthesis and release of prostaglandins by mouse peritoneal macrophages. Prostaglandins (18): 605-610, 1979.
55. Catanzaro A: Suppressor cells in coccidiomycosis. Cell Immunol (64): 235-245, 1981.
56. Kaneene J, Anderson R, Johnson DW, Muscoplat CC: Brucella antigen preparations for in vitro lymphocyte immunostimulation assays for bovine Brucellosis. Infect Immun (22): 486-491, 1978.
57. Dore-Duffy P, Zurier RB: Lymphocyte adherence in multiple sclerosis. Role of monocytes and increased sensitivity of MS lymphocytes to prostaglandin E1. Clin Immunol Immunopathol (19): 303-313, 1981.
58. Wolinsky S, Goodwin JS, Messner RP, Williams RC Jr: Role of prostaglandin in the depressed cell-mediated immune response in rheumatoid arthritis. Clin Immunol Immunopathol (17): 31-36, 1980.
59. Panayi GS, Corrigal V, Youlten LJF: Immunoregulation in the rheumatic diseases. Scand J Rheumatol (38): 9-15, 1980.
60. Chinen Y, Nagaoka K, Sakurami T, Imura H: Depression of lymphocyte blastogenesis in steroid-treated rheumatoid arthritis. Arthritis Rheum (25): 713-717, 1982.
61. Seitz M, Deimann W, Gram N, Hunstein W, Gemsa D: Characterization of blood mononuclear cells of rheumatoid arthritis patients. Clin Immunol Immunopathol (25): 405-416, 1982.
62. Scott PA, Farrell JP: Experimental cutaneous leishmaniasis. J Immunol (127): 2395-2400, 1981.

63. Garin EH, Barratt TM: Effect of indomethacin on lymphocyte response to mitogens in puromycin aminonucleoside nephrosis in the rat. Clin Exp Immunol (49): 639-644, 1982.
64. Kleinhenz ME, Ellner JJ, Spagnuolo PJ, Daniel TM: Suppression of lymphocyte responses by tuberculous plasma and mycobacterial arabinogalactan. J Clin Invest (68): 153-162, 1981.
65. Phung ND, Davidson PT: Increased suppressor cell activity in a patient with mycobacterium avium-intracellular pulmonary disease and hypogammaglobulinemia. Ann Allergy (46): 204-207, 1981.
66. Mason UG, Grenberg LE, Yen SS, Kirkpatrick CH: Indomethacin-response mononuclear cell dysfunction in "atypical" mycobacteriosis. Cell Immunol (71): 54-65, 1982.
67. Koster F, Williams J, Goodwin JS: Specific immunologic unresponsiveness in disseminated Q fever: participation of a T cell--monocyte suppressor circuit. Submitted for publication.
68. Kierszenbaum F: Immunologic deficiency during experimental Chagas' disease (trypanosoma cruzi infection). J Immunol (129): 2202-2205, 1982.
69. Piessens WF, Partono F, Hoffman SL, Ratiwayanto S, Piessens PW, Palmieri JR, Koiman I, Dennis DT, Carney WP: Antigen-specific suppressor T lymphocytes in human lymphatic filariasis. N Engl J Med (307): 144-148, 1982.
70. Goodwin JS, De Horatius R, Israel H, Peake GT, Messner RP: Suppressor cell function in sarcoidosis. Ann Intern Med (90): 169-175, 1979.
71. Rice L, Laughter A, Twomey J: Three suppressor systems in human blood that modulate lymphoproliferation. J Immunol (122): 991-999, 1979.
72. Drysdale B-E, Shin HS: Activation of macrophages for tumor cell cytotoxicity: identification of indomethacin sensitive and insensitive pathways. J Immunol (127): 760-765, 1981.
73. Zighelbolm J, Lichtenstein A, Benjamin D: Response of normal subjects to mitogens: influence of adherent cells. Clin Immunol Immunopathol (19): 406-415, 1981.
74. Metzger A, Hoffeld J, Oppenheim J: Macrophage mediated suppression. J Immunol (124): 983-988, 1980.
75. Lapp WS, Mendes M, Kirchner H, Gemsa D: Prostaglandin synthesis by lymphoid tissue of mice experiencing a graft-versus-host reaction. Cell Immunol (50): 271-281, 1980.
76. Hopkins J, McConnell I, Raniwalla J: Antigen-induced non-specific suppressor factor in sheep efferent lymph is prostaglandin E_2. Immunology (43): 205-210, 1981.
77. Thomas JM, Carver FM, Haisch CE, Fahrenbruch G, Deepe RM, Thomas FT: Suppressor cells in rhesus monkeys treated with antithymocyte globulin. Transplantation (34): 83-89, 1982.
78. Staszak CS, Goodwin JS, Troup GM, Rathak DR, Williams RC Jr: Decreased sensitivity to prostaglandin and histamine in lymphocytes from normal HLA-B12 individuals: a possible role in autoimmunity. J Immunol (125): 181-188, 1980.

79. Kirby PJ, Morley, J, Ponsford JR, MacDonald WI: Defective PGE reactivity in leucocytes of multiple sclerosis patients. Prostaglandins (11): 621-626, 1976.
80. Goodwin JS, Messner RP: Prostaglandin E inhibition of mitogen stimulation in patients with multiple sclerosis. Prostaglandins (15): 281-287, 1978.
81. Dore-Duffy P, Zurier RB: Lymphocyte adherence in multiple sclerosis: effect of aspirin. J Clin Invest (63): 154-159, 1979.
82. Page RC, Clagett JA, Engel LD, Wilde G, Sims T: Effects of prostaglandin on the antigen- and mitogen-driven responses of peripheral blood lymphocytes from patients with adult and juvenile periodonitis. Clin Immunol Immunopathol (11): 77-82, 1978.
83. Goodwin JS, Messner RP: Sensitivity of lymphocytes to prostaglandin E_2 increases in subjects over age 70. J Clin Invest (64): 434-440, 1979.
84. Goodwin JS: Changes in lymphocyte sensitivity to prostaglandin E, histamine, hydrocortisone and x-irradiation with age: studies in a healthy elderly population. Clin Immunol Immunopathol (25): 243-251, 1982.
85. Goodwin JS: Increased sensitivity to prostaglandin E_2 in old people. Prostaglandins Med (3): 395-401, 1979.
86. Delfraissy JF, Garanand P, Wallon C, Balavoine JF, Dormont J: Abolished in vitro antibody response in elderly: exclusive involvement of prostaglandin-induced T suppressor cells. Clin Immunol Immunopathol (24): 377-385, 1982.
87. Ceuppens J, Goodwin JS: Endogenous prostaglandin E_2 enhances polyclonal immunoglobulin production by tonically inhibiting T suppressor cell activity. Cell Immunol (70): 41-54, 1982.
88. Goldberg EH, Frikke MJ: The role of suppressor cells in the fetal escape of maternal immunologic rejection. In: Goodwin JS (ed) Suppressor cells in human disease. Marcel Dekker, New York, 1981, pp 247-266.
89. Olding LB, Benirschke K, Oldstone M: Inhibition of mitosis of lymphocytes from human adults by lymphocytes from human newborns. Clin Immunol Immunopathol (3): 79-88, 1974.
90. Olding LB, Oldstone M: Thymus-derived peripheral lymphocytes from human newborns inhibit division of their mother's lymphocytes. J Immunol (116): 682-687, 1976.
91. Johnsen S, Olding LB, Westberg NG, Wilhelmsson L: Strong suppression by mononuclear leukocytes from human newborns on material leukocytes: mediation by prostaglandins. Clin Immunol Immunopathol (23): 606-615, 1982.
92. Goodwin JS, Messner RP, Peake GT: Increased sensitivity of maternal lymphocytes to PGE_2. Clin Res (26): 514A, 1978.
93. Vanderbeeken Y, Vlieghe MP, Delespesse G: Regulation of the lymphocyte response to phytohemagglutinin during pregnancy: role of adherent cells and prostaglandins. Am J Reproduct Immunol (1): 233-235, 1981.

94. Goodwin JS, Bromberg S, Staszak C, Kaszubowski PA, Messner RP, Neal JF: Effect of physical stress on sensitivity of lymphocytes to inhibition by prostaglandin E_2. J Immunol (127): 518-522, 1981.
95. Wang BS, Heacock EH, Mannick JA: Characterization of suppressor cells generated in mice after surgical trauma. Clin Immunol Immunopathol (24): 161-170, 1982.
96. Hasler F, Bluestein HG, Zvaifler NJ, Epstein LB: Analysis of the defects responsible for the impaired regulation of EBV-induced B cell proliferation by rheumatoid arthritis lymphocytes. J Immunol (131): 768-772, 1983.
97. Goodwin JS, Ceuppens JL, Rodriguez MA: Effect of nonsteroidal antiinflammatory agents on immunologic function in patients with rheumatoid arthritis. J Am Med Assoc (250): 2485-2489, 1983.
98. Ceuppens JL, Goodwin JS: Non-steroidal anti-inflammatory agents inhibit the synthesis of IgM rheumatoid factor in vitro. Lancet (1): 528-533, 1982.
99. Kelly RH, Miller DH, Rodnan GP, Hagmann J: Prostaglandin-mediated inhibition of lymphokine secretion in normal individuals and patients with progressive systemic sclerosis (scleroderma, PSS). Agents Actions (12): 471-477, 1982.
100. Taffet S, Russell SW: Macrophage-mediated tumor cell killing: regulation of expression of cytolytic activity by prostaglandin E. J Immunol (126): 424-429, 1981.
101. Goodwin JS, Bankhurst AD, Murphy S, Selinger DS, Messner RP, Williams RC Jr: Partial reversal of the cellular immune defect in common variable immunodeficiency with indomethacin. J Clin Lab Immunol (1): 197-204,1978.
102. Muscoplat CC, Rakich PM, Thoen CO, Johnson DW: Enhancement of lymphocyte blastogenic and delayed hypersensitivity skin responses by indomethacin. Infect Immun (20): 627-632, 1978.
103. Lipsmeyer E: Effect of cimetidine and indomethacin on delayed hypersensitivity. Transplantation (33): 107-113, 1982.
104. Anderson CB, Jaffee BM, Graff RJ: Prolongation of murine skin allografts by prostaglandin E_1. Transplantation (23): 444-449, 1977.
105. Blyth WA, Hill TJ, Field HJ, Harbour DA: Reactivation of herpes simplex virus infection of prostaglandins. J Gen Virol (33): 547-551, 1976.
106. Tracey DE, Adkinson NF: Prostaglandin synthesis inhibitors potentiate the BCG-induced augmentation of natural killer cell activity. J Immunol (125): 136-141, 1980.
107. Goodwin JS, Selinger DS, Messner RP, Reed WP: Effect of indomethacin in vivo on humoral and cellular immunity in humans. Infect Immun (19): 430-437, 1978.
108. Grohmann P, Porzsolt F, Quirt I, Miller R, Phillips R: Stimulation of human NK cell activity by cultured cells. Clin Exp Immunol (44): 611-614, 1981.

109. Palmer DG, Barbezat GO, Gibbins BL, Grennan DM, Lum J, Myers DB, Wilson K: A single-blind crossover trial of the anti-inflammatory drug sodium meclofenamate and placebo, including an evaluation of hand grip and of lymphocyte responsiveness. Curr Med Res Opin (7): 359-367, 1981.
110. Palmer DG, Ferry DG, Gibbins BL, Hall SM, Grennan DM, Lum J, Myers DB: Ibuprofen and diflunisal in rheumatoid arthritis: a double-blind comparative trial. NZ Med J (94): 45-47, 1981.
111. Bach MA, Fournier C, Bach JF: Regulation of theta-antigen expression by agents altering cyclic AMP level and by thymic factor. Ann NY Acad Sci (249): 316-320, 1975.
112. Gualde N, Rigaud M, Bach JF: Stimulation of prostaglandin synthesis by the serum factor (FTS). Cell Immunol (70): 362-366, 1982.
113. Rinaldi-Garaci C, Del Gobbo V, Favalli C, Garaci E, Bistoni F, Jaffe BM: Induction of serum thymic-like activity in adult thymectomized mice by a synthetic analog of PGE_2. Cell Immunol (72): 97-101, 1982.
114. Burchiel SW, Warner NL: Cyclic AMP modulation of Fc receptor expression on a pre-B cell lymphoma. J Immunol (124): 1016-1021, 1980.
115. Offner H, Danneskiold-Samsoe B, Dore-Duffy P: Effect of prostaglandins and aspirin on active E-rosette formation in patients with multiple sclerosis. Clin Immunol Immunopathol (22): 159-165, 1982.
116. Stobo JD, Kennedy MS, Goldyne ME: Prostaglandin E modulation of the mitogenic response of human T cells. J Clin Invest (64): 1188-1192, 1979.
117. Gualde N, Goodwin JS: Effects of prostaglandin E_2 and preincubation on lectin-stimulated proliferation of human T cell subsets. Cell Immunol (70): 373-378, 1982.
118. Kendall R, Targan S: The dual effect of prostaglandin and ethanol on the natural killer cytolytic process. J Immunol (125): 2770-2777, 1980.
119. Schultz RM, Pavlidis NA, Stylos WA, Chirigos MA: Regulation of macrophage tumoricidal function: a role for prostaglandins of the E series. Science (202): 320-327, 1978.
120. McCarthy ME, Zwilling BS: Differential effects of prostaglandins on the antitumor activity of normal and BCG-activated macrophages. Cell Immunol (60): 91-97, 1981.
121. Schnyder J, Dewald B, Baggiolini M: Effects of cyclooxygenase inhibitors and prostaglandin E_2 macrophage activation in vitro. Prostaglandins (22): 411-416, 1979.
122. Razin E, Bauminger S, Globerson A: Effect of prostaglandins on phagocytes of sheep erythrocytes by mouse peritoneal macrophages. J Reticuloendothel Soc (23): 237-242, 1978.
123. Wahl LM, Olsen CE, Wahl SM, McCarthy JB, Sandberg AL, Mergenhagen SE: Prostaglandin and cyclic AMP regulation of macrophage involvement in connective tissue destruction. Ann NY Acad Sci (332): 271-278, 1979.

124. Smith JW, Steiner AL, Parker CW: Human lymphocytic metabolism. Effects of cyclic and noncyclic nucleotides on stimulation by phytohemagglutinin. J Clin Invest (50): 442-449, 1971.
125. Melmon KL, Bourne HR, Weinstein Y, Shearer GM, Kram J, Bauminger S: Separation of specific antibody-forming mouse cells by their adherence to insolubilized endogenous hormones. J Clin Invest (53): 22-27, 1974.
126. Goodwin JS, Wiik A, Lewis M, Bankhurst AD, Williams RC Jr: High affinity binding sites for prostaglandin E on human lymphocytes. Cell Immunol (43): 150-159, 1979.
127. Kalmar L, Gergely P: Enhancement of mitogen-induced lymphocyte proliferation after preincubation is due to altered sensitivity to prostaglandins. Immunol Lett (4): 179-183, 1982.
128. Goodwin JS, Bromberg S, Messner RP: Studies on the cyclic AMP response to prostaglandin in human lymphocytes. Cell Immunol (60): 298-307, 1981.
129. Webb DR, Rogers TJ, Ong S, Steiner A: Detection of prostaglandin induced antigen-stimulated changes in splenic AMP levels by immunofluorescence. Prostaglandins Med (5): 141-147, 1980.
130. Goodwin JS, Kaszubowski PA, Williams RC Jr: Cyclic adenosine monophosphate response to prostaglandin E2 in subpopulations of human lymphocytes. J Exp Med (150): 1260-1267, 1979.
131. Moretta L, Webb SR, Grossi CE, Lydyard PM, Cooper MD: Functional analysis of two human T-cell subpopulations: help and suppression of B-cell responses by T-cells bearing receptors for IgM or IgG. J Exp Med (146): 184-200, 1977.
132. Pelus C, Bockman R: Increased prostaglandin synthesis by microphages from tumor bearing mice. J Immunol (123): 2118-2124, 1979.
133. Glaser M: Indomethacin-sensitive suppressor cells regulate the cell-mediated cytotoxic response to SV 40-induced tumor-associated antigens in mice. Eur J Immunol (10): 489-496, 1980.
134. Goodwin JS, Messner RP, Bankhurst AD, Peake GT, Saiki JH, Williams RC Jr: Prostaglandin-producing suppressor cells in Hodgkin's disease. N Engl J Med (197): 263-269, 1977.
135. Bockman RS: Stage dependent reduction in T-colony formation in Hodgkin's disease. J Clin Invest (66): 523-531, 1980.
136. DeShazo RP: Indomethacin-responsive mononuclear cell dysfunction in Hodgkin's disease. Clin Immunol Immunopathol (17): 66-72, 1980.
137. Sibbitt WL Jr, Bankhurst AD, Williams RC Jr: Studies of cell subpopulations mediating mitogen hyporesponsiveness in patients with Hodgkin's disease. J Clin Invest (61): 55-63, 1978.
138. Johnsen SA: Prostaglandin associated immunosuppression. Doctoral thesis, University of Gateborg, Sweden, 1983.
139. Bankhurst AD, Kauffman G, Goodwin JS, Williams RC Jr: Suppressor leukocytes in anergic patients with solid tumors. J Lab Clin Immunol (3): 3-10, 1980.

140. Vosixa G, Thies J: Effect of indomethacin on blastogenesis of lymphocytes from cancer patients: differentiation of patient types. Clin Immunol Immunopathol (13): 30-36, 1979.
141. Maca RD, Panje W: Indomethacin sensitive suppressor cell activity in head and neck cancer patients pre and post irradiation therapy. Cancer (50): 438-489, 1982.
142. Balch CM, Dougherty PA, Tilden A: Excessive prostaglandin E_2 production by suppressor monocytes in head and neck cancer patients. Ann Surg (196): 645-650, 1982.
143. Braun DP, Harris JE: Relationship of leukocyte numbers, immunoregulatory cell function, and phytohemagglutinin responsiveness in cancer patients. J Natl Cancer Inst (67): 809-814, 1981.
144. Klein DC, Raisl LG: Prostaglandins: stimulation of bone resorption in tissue culture. Endocrinology (86): 1436-1443, 1970.
145. Bennett A, Del Tacca M, Stamford IF, Zebro T: Prostaglandins from tumours of human large bowel. Br J Cancer (35): 881-884, 1977.
146. Cummings KB, Robertson RP: Prostaglandin: increased production by renal cell carcinoma. J Urol (118): 720-727, 1977.
147. Husby G, Strickland RG, Rigler GL, Peake GT, Williams RC Jr: Direct immunochemical detection of prostaglandin E and cyclic nucleotides in human malignant tumors. Cancer (40): 1629-1636, 1977.
148. Powles TJ, Coomes RC, Neville AM, Ford HT, Gazet JC, Levine L: 15-keto-13, 14 dihydroprostaglandin E2 concentrations in serum of patients with breast cancer. Lancet (2): 138-143, 1977.
149. Rolland PH, Martin PM, Jacquemier J, Rolland AM, Toga M: Prostaglandin in human breast cancer: evidence suggesting that an elevated prostaglandin production is a marker of high metastatic potential for neoplastic cells. J Natl Cancer Inst (64): 1061-1068, 1980.
150. Sykes JAC, Maddox IS: Prostaglandin production by experimental tumours and effects of anti-inflammatory compounds. Nature New Biology (237): 59-61, 1972.
151. Tashjian AH, Voelkel EF, Levine L, Goldhaber P: Evidence that the bone-resorption stimulating factor produced by mouse fibrosarcoma cells is prostaglandin. J Exp Med (136): 1329-1336, 1972.
152. Owen K, Gomolka D, Droller MJ: Lymphocyte induced production of prostaglandin E2 by tumor cells in vitro: requirements for direct contact and lymphocyte viability. Cell Immunol (55): 428-435, 1980.
153. Plescia OJ, Smith AH, Grinwich K: Subversion of immune system by tumor cells and role of prostaglandins. Proc Natl Acad Sci (72): 1848-1854, 1975.
154. Grinwich KD, Plescia OJ: Tumor-mediated immunosuppression: prevention by inhibitors of prostaglandin synthesis. Prostaglandins (14): 1175-1183, 1977.

155. Hial V, Horakova Z, Shaff FE, Beaven MA: Alteration of tumor growth by aspirin and indomethacin: studies with two transplantable tumors in mouse. Eur J Pharmacol (37): 367-376, 1976.
156. Lynch NR, Casatles M, Astonin M, Salomon JC: Mechanism of inhibition of tumor growth by aspirin and indomethacin. Br J Cancer (38): 503-509, 1978.
157. Humes JL, Cupo J, Strausser, HR: Effects of indomethacin on Moloney sarcoma virus-induced tumors. Prostaglandins (6): 463-469, 1974.
158. Strausser HR, Humes JL: Prostaglandin synthesis inhibition: effect on bone changes and sarcoma tumor induction in mice. Int J Cancer (15): 724-729, 1975.
159. Bennett A, Houghton J, Leaper DJ, Stamford IF: Cancer growth, response to treatment and survival time in mice: beneficial effect of the prostaglandin synthesis inhibitor flurbiprofen. Prostaglandins (17): 179-191, 1979.
160. Pollard M, Luckert, PH: Effect of indomethacin on intestinal tumors induced in rats by the acetate derivative of dimethylnitrosamine. Science (214): 558-559, 1981.
161. Waddell WR, Gerner RE, Reich MD: Nonsteroid antiinflammatory drugs for desmoid tumors and carcinoma of the stomach, submitted for publication, 1982.
162. Panje WR: Regression of head and neck carcinoma with a prostaglandin synthesis inhibitor. Arch Otolaryngol (107): 658-663, 1981.
163. Galasko CSB, Bennett A: A relationship of bone distinction in skeletal metastases to osteoclast activation and prostaglandins. Nature (263): 508-513, 1976.
164. Powles TJ, Clar SA, Easty DM, Easty CG, Neville AM: The inhibition by aspirin and indomethacin of osteolytic tumor deposits and hypercalcaemia in rats with Walker tumour, and its possible application to human breast cancer. Br J Cancer (28): 316-321, 1973.
165. Yoneda R, Mundy GR: Prostaglandins are necessary for osteoclast-activating factor production by activated peripheral blood leukocytes. J Exp Med (149): 279-288, 1979.
166. Lupulescu A: Enhancement of carcinogenesis by prostaglandins in male, albino Swiss mice. J Natl Cancer Inst (61): 97-103, 1978.
167. Levine L, Ohucki K: Retinoids as well as tumor promoters enhance deacylation of cellular lipids and prostaglandin production in MDCK cells. Nature (276): 274-280, 1978.
168. Ohuchi K, Levine L: Stimulation of prostaglandin synthesis by tumor-promoting phorbol-12-13-diesters in canine kidney (MDCK) cells. J Biol Chem (253): 4783-4790, 1978.
169. Yamasaki H, Mufson RA, Weinstein IB: Phorbol ester induced prostaglandin synthesis and [3H]-TPA metabolism by TPA-sensitive and TPA-resistant friend erythroleukemia cells. Biochem Biophys Res Commun (89): 1018-1025, 1979.
170. Buick RN, Fry SE, Salmon SE: Effect of host-cell interactions on clonogenic carcinoma cells in human malignant effusions. Br J Cancer (41): 695-704, 1980.

171. Santoro MG, Philpott GW, Jaffe BM: Inhibition of tumor growth in vivo and in vitro by prostaglandin E. Nature (263): 777-779, 1976.
172. Stringfellow D, Fitzpatrick F: Prostaglandin Dα controls pulmonary metastasis of malignant melanoma cells. Nature (282): 76-84, 1979.
173. Favalli C, Garaci E, Etheredge E, Santoro MG, Jaffe BM: Influence of PGE in the immune response in melanoma-bearing mice. J Immunol (125): 897-906, 1980.
174. Hofer D, Dubitsky AM, Reilly P, Santoro MG, Jaffe BM: The interactions between indomethacin and cytotoxic drugs in mice bearing B-16 melanomas. Prostaglandins (20): 1033-1038, 1980.
175. Santoro MG, Jaffe, BM: Inhibition of friend erythroleukemia-cell tumors in vivo by a synthetic analogue of prostaglandin E2. Br J Cancer (39): 408-413, 1979.
176. Karmali RA, Horrobin DF, Menenzes J, Patel P: The relationship between concentrations of prostaglandin A1, E1, E2 and E2 alpha and rates of cell proliferation. Pharmacol Res Commun (11): 69-76, 1979.
177. Klimpel GR: Soluble factors from BCG-induced suppressor cells inhibit in vitro PFC responses but not cytotoxic responses. Cell Immunol (47): 218-226, 1979.
178. Klimpel G, Henney CS: BCG-induced suppressor cells. I. Demonstration of a macrophage-like suppressor cell that inhibits cytotoxic T-cell generation in vitro. J Immunol (120): 563-570, 1978.
179. Klimpel GR, Okada M, Henney CS: Inhibition of in vitro cytotoxic responses by BCG-induced microphage-like suppressor cells. II. Suppression occurs at the level of 'helper' T cell. J Immunol (123): 350-357, 1979.
180. Neta R, Slavin, SB: Adjuvants in the induction of suppressor cells. Infect Immun (23): 360-365, 1979.
181. Savary CA, Lotzova E: Suppression of natural killer cell cytotoxicity by splenocytes from corynebacterium parvum-injected bone marrow-tolerant and infant mice. J Immunol (120): 239-245, 1978.
182. Grimm W, Seitz M, Kirchner H, Gemsa D: Prostaglandin synthesis in spleen cell cultures of mice injected with corynebacterium parvum. Cell Immunol (40): 419-426, 1978.
183. Wahl SM, Wahl LM, McCarthy JB, Chedid L, Mergenhagen SE: Macrophage activation by mycobacterial water soluble compounds and synthetic maramyl dipeptide. J Immunol (122): 2226-2232, 1979.
184. Lynch NR, Salomon J-C: Tumor growth inhibition and potentiation of immunotherapy by indomethacin in mice. J Natl Cancer Inst (62): 117-121, 1979.
185. Droller M, Gomolka D: Interferon expression and prostaglandin synthetase inhibition in the in vitro and in vivo manipulation of immune response expression in an animal model of bladder cancer. Cell Immunol (72): 1-13, 1982.

186. Droller MA, Gomolka D: Inhibition of tumor growth in association with modification of in vivo immune response by indomethacin and polyinosinic-polycytidylic acid. Cancer Res (42): 5038-5045, 1982.
187. Goodwin JS, Webb DR: Regulation of the immune response by prostaglandins. Clin Immunol Immunopathol (15): 106-122, 1980.
188. Goodwin JS, Ceuppens J: Regulation of the immune response by prostaglandins. J Clin Immunol (3): 295-305, 1984.

Chapter 2

PROSTAGLANDINS AND EXPRESSION OF LYMPHOCYTE CYTOTOXICITY

Michael J. Droller

INTRODUCTION

The suggestion that prostaglandins may play an important role in immune response/tumor cell interactions is based upon several observations. First, a variety of prostaglandins are produced both by cells that are themselves active in the expression and regulation of immune response activity (1-4) as well as by a number of tumor targets (5,6). Second, the production of prostaglandins has been found to increase as a result of direct contact between effector lymphocytes and tumor targets (7). Third, prostaglandins at levels produced during these interactions have been shown to influence the ultimate expression in vitro of lymphocyte and macrophage cytotoxicity against tumor targets (8-12).

Interpretations of such observations have led to two major conclusions. First, prostaglandins may induce certain functions of cellular immune response activity, (2,13,14), at the same time regulate the extent of other aspects of immune response expression (8-12), and ultimately restore immunologic homeostasis. Second, tumor cell prostaglandin production, by inhibiting lymphocyte and macrophage activity, may actually subvert the putative immune response mounted against them (11,15).

These interpretations prompted us to explore the role of prostaglandins in several tumor systems. It soon became apparent that the interactions initially suspected to be straightforward were actually far more complex. They still remain largely undefined. The present details the directions we have followed and our observations to date.

OBSERVATIONS

Initially, we examined a variety of human tumor cell lines that had been maintained in monolayer by serial passage for many years. These included T_{24} (transitional cell epithelial tumor), HCV_{29} (normal bladder transitional cell epithelium), and MANO (colon carcinoma). Each of these

J.S. Goodwin (ed.), PROSTAGLANDINS AND IMMUNITY.

cell lines produced prostaglandin E_2 and F_2 , as determined by radioimmunoassay, but not prostaglandin I_2, as determined by the inhibitory activity of cell supernates on platelet aggregation (11) (Fig. 1A, B).

When purified peripheral blood lymphocytes from human volunteers were placed on confluent tumor cell monolayers, the production of prostaglandin E_2 by these tumor cells was markedly increased (11). The amounts of these increments varied. With T_{24}, levels were 5-10 times as high as when tumor cells were incubated alone; with HCV_{29} and MANO, levels were only two-three times as high. Prostaglandin E_2 production by lymphocytes incubated alone under identical test conditions were negligible (11).

In related studies, prostaglandin E_2 at concentrations similar to those produced by the tumor cells induced the accumulation of intracellular cyclic AMP in peripheral blood lymphocytes (11). Earlier studies had shown that intracellular cyclic AMP in lymphocytes and in macrophages was associated with inhibition of cytotoxicity (16,17). Moreover, blastogenesis, cell activation, and production of cytotoxic materials by these cells had also been found to be inhibited (18-20).

These observations suggested that prostaglandin production by tumor cells might be a factor in limiting the capacity of the host to effect an immune response to neoplasia. Moreover, that the highest levels of prostaglandins were produced upon exposure to effector lymphocytes suggested that such a defense mechanism by tumor cells, expressed at a time of greatest challenge to tumor cell survival, would be expected to be highly effective (11).

An in vitro cytotoxicity assay in which lymphocytes were incubated with ^{51}Chromium-labelled tumor target cells was used to confirm these suggestions. Prostaglandins E_1 and E_2 at concentrations produced by tumor cells were found to inhibit both natural and antibody-dependent lymphocyte cytotoxicity directed against these targets (21) (Figs 2 and 3). Addition of theophylline (a phosphodiesterase inhibitor) to these samples demonstrated further inhibition of lymphocyte cytotoxicity by both natural killer and antibody-dependent mechanisms (11,21). This was thought to reflect the increased accumulation of cyclic AMP brought about by prostaglandin-induced cyclic AMP production in association with theophylline-induced inhibition of cyclic AMP metabolism.

Preincubation of lymphocytes with varying concentrations of prostaglandins E_1 and E_2 prior to their addition to the target cells

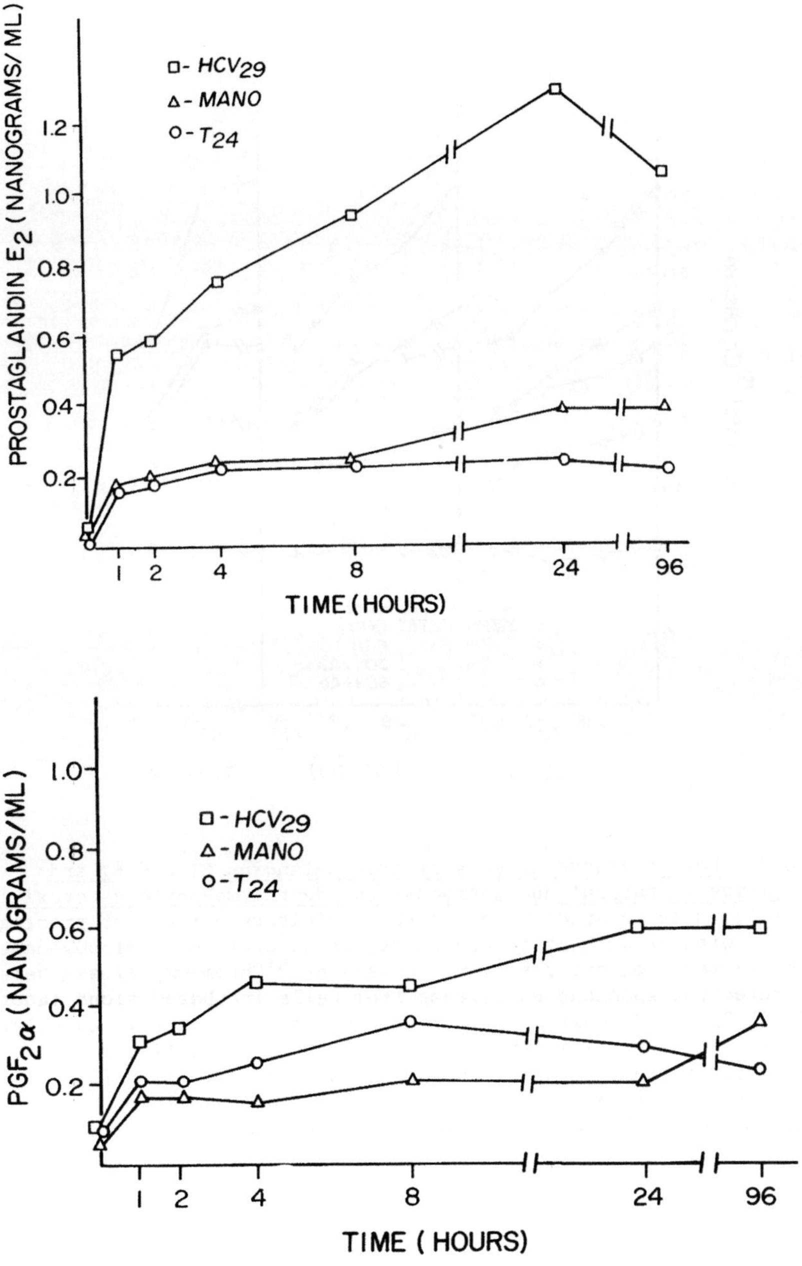

Figure 1A, B. Production of prostaglandin E_2 and $F_{2\alpha}$ by tumor cells incubated with arachidonic acid in vitro.

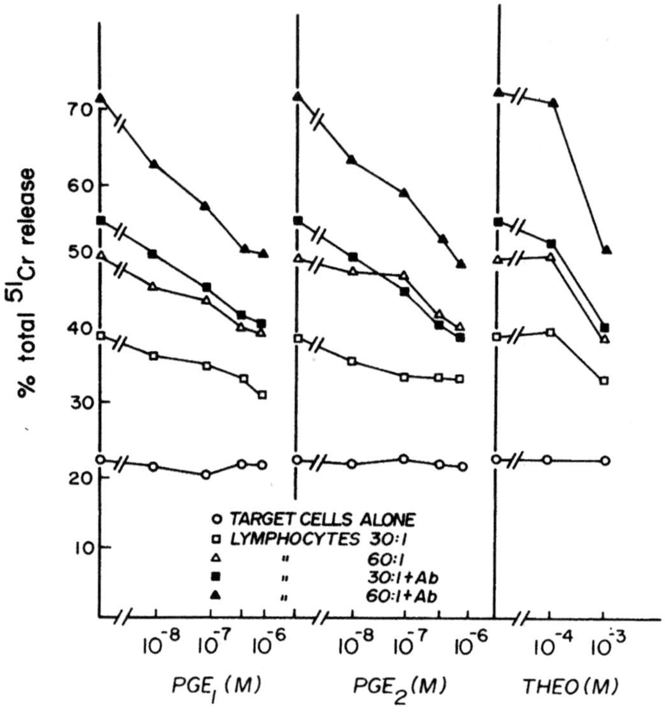

Figure 2. Dose response effects of prostaglandins E1 and E2 and theophylline on natural and antibody-dependent lymphocyte cytotoxicity against T24. These studies tested the inhibitory effects of prostaglandins E_1 and E_2 with or without theophylline, on natural and antibody-dependent lymphocyte-mediated cytotoxicity. Levels of ^{51}Chromium-release were uncorrected for spontaneous release from cells incubated alone (approximately 20-25%). Incubation time at 37° C was 16-20 hours. Calculations were based on ^{51}Chromium levels in supernatants and pellets: % ^{51}Chromium = $\{cpm_{supernate}/(cpm_{supernate} + cpm_{pellet})\} \times 100$. Results are expressed as the average of duplicate samples {Reproduced from (21) with permission of Academic Press}

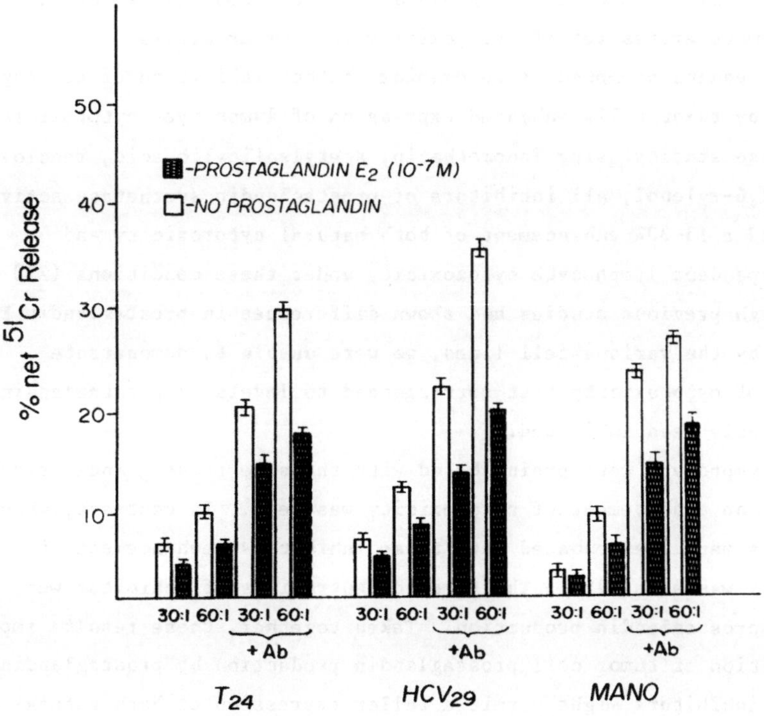

Figure 3. Effect of prostaglandin E_2 on lymphocyte natural and antibody-dependent cytotoxicity against tumor targets. Using a cytotoxicity assay identical to that described in the preceding figure, lymphocytes at 30:1 or 60:1 effector cell:target cell ratio were tested for cytotoxicity either with or without antibody (Ab) against T_{24}, HCV_{29}, or MANO tumor targets. Parallel samples contained prostaglandin E_2 at 10^{-7}M final concentration. Results are expressed as the mean of triplicate samples +/- 1 S.E.

produced similar inhibition of both antibody-dependent and natural lymphocyte cytotoxicity (21). In contrast, preincubation of tumor target cells did not effect ultimate expression of cytotoxicity in similar assays.

These results prompted us to examine whether inhibition of prostaglandin production by tumor cells enhanced expression of lymphocyte cytotoxicity. Dose response studies using indomethacin, acetylsalicylic acid, fenclozic acid, and 2,6-xylenol, all inhibitors of prostaglandin synthetase activity, demonstrated a 15-30% enhancement of both natural cytotoxicity and antibody-dependent lymphocyte cytotoxicity under these conditions (22) (Fig 5). Although previous studies had shown differences in prostaglandin E_2 production by the various cell lines, we were unable to demonstrate increments of cytotoxicity that corresponded to levels of prostaglandin that had presumeably been inhibited.

When lymphocyte were preincubated with the same prostaglandin synthetase inhibitors, no enhancement of cytotoxicity was seen. In contrast, when tumor target cells were preincubated with these inhibitors, enhancement of cytotoxicity was seen (22). The same concentrations of inhibitor were found to prevent prostaglandin production. Taken together, these results implied that inhibition of tumor cell prostaglandin production by prostaglandin synthetase inhibitors might permit a fuller expression of both natural and antibody-dependent cytotoxicity in these systems.

In order to ascertain the applicability of these observations in vivo, we initiated studies in an animal model of carcinogen-induced bladder cancer. Initially, we sought to determine whether tumor cells in this animal model produced prostaglandins, and what conditions effected such production. Tumor targets were derived from a carcinogen-induced bladder cancer (23). Addition of purified splenic or peripheral blood lymphocytes from Fischer rats to monolayers of these tumor cells induced prostaglandin E_2 production, as determined by radioimmunoassay (24) (Fig. 6). Dose response increments in prostaglandin production coincided with the addition of increasing numbers of effector cells to the tumor cells (24). No prostaglandins were produced by tumor cells after exposure to thymus or lymph node lymphocytes in these assays, suggesting that prostaglandin production was largely a response to effector cell exposure.

Irradiation or sonication of lymphocytes prior to their addition to tumor cells led to lower levles of prostaglandin production (7), suggesting that effector lymphocytes had to be viable to induce prostaglandin

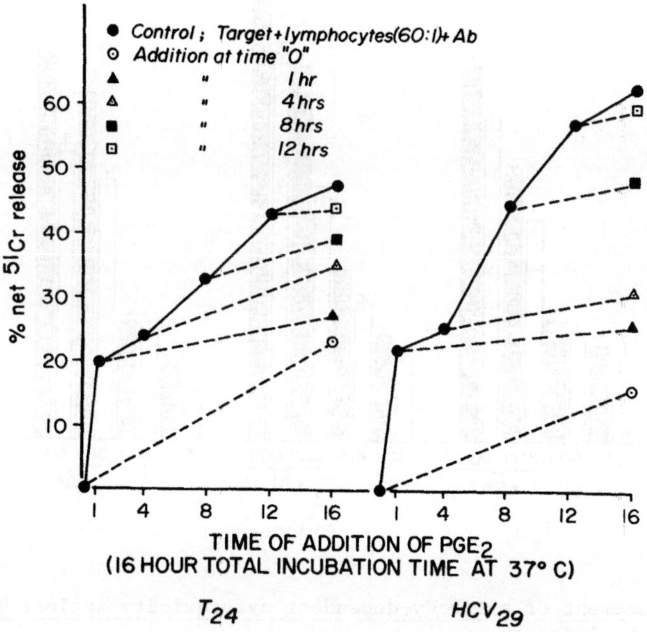

Figure 4. Time course of effect of prostaglandin E_2 on antibody-dependent lymphocyte cytotoxicity. At various times after the onset of incubation at 37° C, prostaglandin E_2 at 10^{-7}M final concentration was added to assay tubes containing lymphocytes and ^{51}Chromium-labelled T_{24} target cells at a 60:1 ratio and anti-T_{24} antiserum at 10^{-6} dilution. At the same time intervals supernates and pellets were processed for the determination of ^{51}Chromium release in parallel tubes to which no prostaglandin had been added. Incubation of tubes receiving prostaglandin was continued for a total of 16-20 hours before processing. Per cent ^{51}Chromium-release in all samples was corrected for spontaneous release from target cells incubated alone (14-20%). Those samples connected by the solid line in this figure represent tubes which received no prostaglandin that were assayed for ^{51}Chromium-release at the times indicated. Each symbol in this line is connected by a broken line to a companion symbol which represents tubes to which prostaglandin E_2 was added at that particular time but which were then further incubated for a total of 16-20 hours before determination of ^{51}Chromium-release.
{Reproduced from (21) with permission of Academic Press}

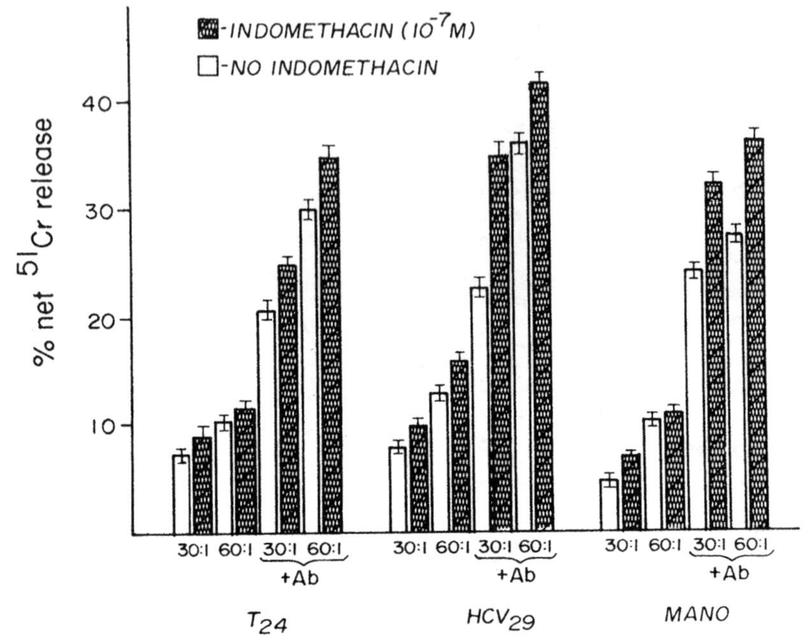

Figure 5. Enhancement of antibody-dependent cytotoxicity against T_{24}, HCV_{29}, and MANO by indomethacin.

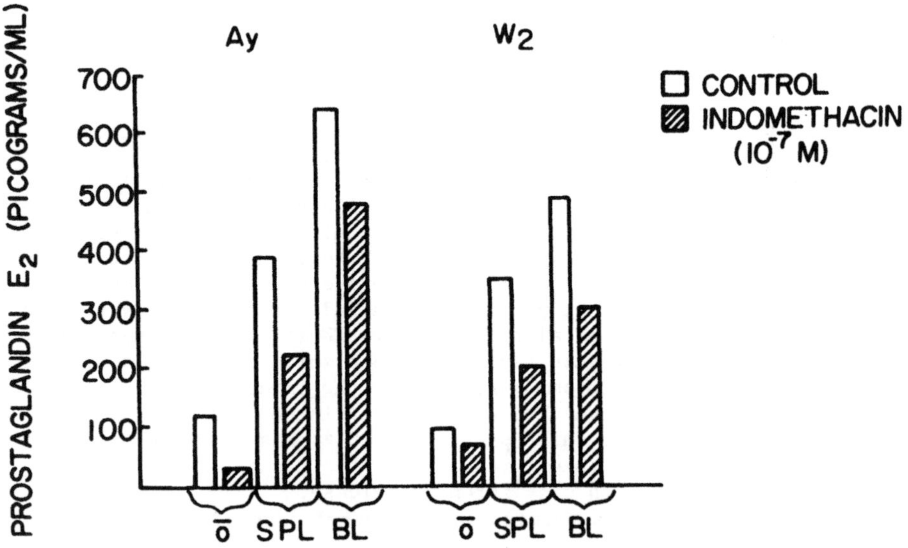

Figure 6. Comparison of effects of blood versus splenic lymphocytes on tumor cell prostaglandin E_2 production by rat cell lines Ay and W_2. {Reproduced from (24) with permission of Waverly Press}

production. In addition, when lymphocytes were added on a platform overlying the tumor monolayers so that direct contact was prevented, less prostaglandin production occurred. When the same lymphocytes were then layered directly onto fresh tumor cell monolayers, prostaglandin production was again seen (7). This suggested a requirement for direct contact between functionally active effector cells and tumor target cells for prostaglandin production to occur.

Next, we thought it important to characterize more accurately the type of prostaglandin produced under these circumstances. To this end, bladder tumor cells, purified splenic lymphocytes, and peritoneal exudate cells were labelled with ^{14}C-dihomo-γ-linoleic acid or ^{14}C-arachidonic acid (precursors of prostaglandins E_1 and E_2 respectively). Labelled effector cells were then incubated with unlabelled tumor cells and unlabelled effector cells were incubated with labelled tumor cells. Supernates and cell pellets were separately extracted and assayed for prostaglandin production using thin layer silica gel chromatography.

Peritoneal exudate cells were found to produce prostaglandin E_2 when incubated together with unlabelled tumor target cells (Fig 7). No prostaglandin E_1 was produced under identical circumstances. Prelabelled tumor cells also produced prostaglandin E_2, (but no prostaglandin E_1) when unlabelled effector cells were added to them (Fig 8). The highest levels of prostaglandins were produced by peritoneal exudate cells. Minimal levels were produced by effector splenic lymphocytes alone.

These observations were applied in an examination of the effects of manipulation of prostaglandin production on immune response expression and possible inhibition of tumor growth both in vitro and in vivo. In initial experiments, addition of prostaglandins E_1 and E_2 to cytotoxicity assays inhibited natural cytotoxicity by splenic lymphocytes against bladder tumor cells in a dose-response fashion. However, addition of macrophages to lymphocytes in parallel assay samples failed to inhibit cytotoxicity by effector lymphocytes, even though macrophages had been shown to produce substantial amounts of prostaglandins. Addition of indomethacin to the same samples failed to alter levels of cytotoxicity by lymphocytes alone or by lymphocytes in the presence of macrophages (25).

Negative results were also obtained in attempts to manipulate the prostaglandin system in vivo (26). Inoculation of tumor-bearing or control animals with indomethacin failed to alter levels of lymphocyte cytotoxicity

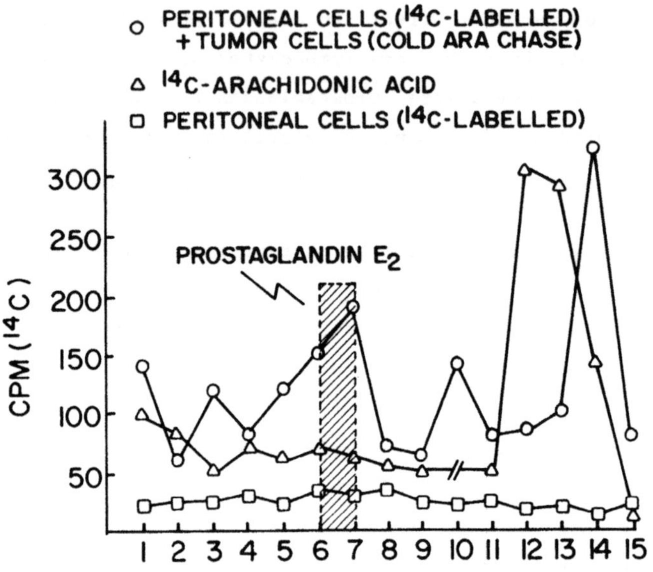

Figure 7. Prostaglandin E_2 production by ^{14}C-arachidonic acid-labelled peritoneal exudate cells.

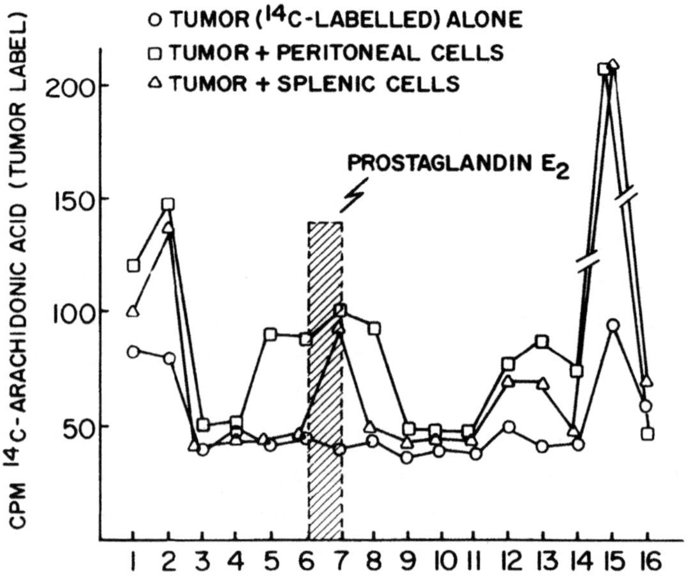

Figure 8. Prostaglandin E_2 production by tumor cells labelled with ^{14}C-arachidonic acid.

seen in subsequent in vitro assays (Fig 9). In these studies, splenic lymphocytes from tumor-bearing animals generally expressed lower levels of cytotoxicity than did lymphocytes from control animals. Indomethacin failed to effect these differences. Similar negative findings characterized the effect of in vivo indomethacin on cytotoxicity by peritoneal macrophages either alone or when added to lymphocytes in in vitro assays.

Though enhancement of natural cytotoxicity occurred in vitro in response to interferon in the same bladder tumor model, addition of indomethacin to these samples depressed rather than stimulated otherwise enhanced levels of cytotoxicity (26). Macrophages did not appear to effect these interactions since indomethacin in vitro did not enhance their cytotoxicity in response to interferon either in the presence or absence of splenic lymphocytes. No toxic effects of indomethacin could be detected.

In vivo treatment of tumor-bearing animals with indomethacin appeared in initial experiments to inhibit tumor growth in a carcinogen-induced model of bladder cancer. Correlations with enhanced lymphocyte or macrophage cytotoxicity, however, were not observed (27). When a transplantable model of bladder cancer was examined, initial inhibition of tumor growth by indomethacin was also seen (28). After therapy was discontinued, minimal or no ultimate inhibitory effect on tumor growth by indomethacin could be appreciated. Correspondingly, expression of macrophage and/or lymphocyte cytotoxicity in this system did not appear to be effected. Only in certain instances in which higher concentrations of indomethacin were used did an enhancement effect on macrophage/lymphocyte cytotoxicity become evident (26).

Polyinosinic.polycytidylic acid (poly I:C), an inducer of interferon, was consistently found to inhibit tumor growth and enhance lymphocyte and macrophage cytotoxicity in these systems (27,28) (Fig 10). The effect of indomethacin in these samples, however, was inhibitory rather than stimulatory, even when macrophages were present during cytotoxicity testing. Although concomitant treatment with indomethacin in these animals led to further inhibition of tumor growth, lower levels of natural cytotoxicity were seen than when lymphocytes from animals treated with poly I:C alone were examined. In vitro addition of either indomethacin and/or interferon to parallel cytotoxicity samples containing lymphocytes or macrophages alone, or combinations of the two, did not demonstrate the cellular immunologic mechanism by which tumor growth appeared to have been inhibited. In addition, although effects of poly I:C on tumor growth and lymphocyte

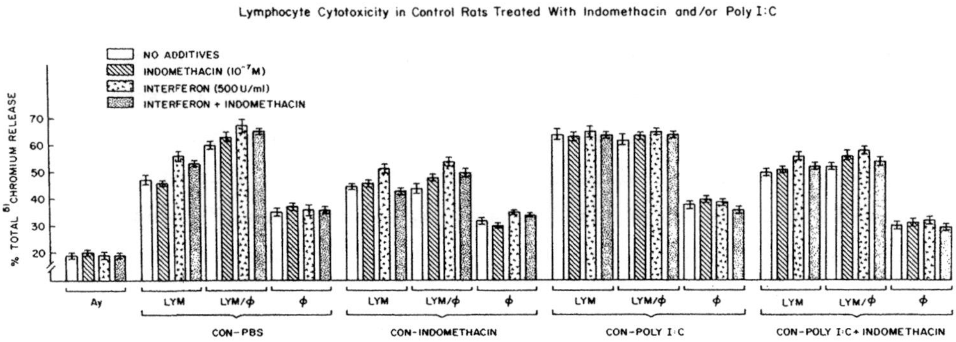

Figure 9. Lymphocyte/macrophage cytotoxicity in control rats treated in vivo with indomethacin and/or poly I:C. Control rats were treated intraperitoneally either with phosphate buffered saline (PBS), indomethacin (INDO), poly I:C, or the combination of poly I:C and indomethacin in every other day for 5 treatments. Splenic lymphocytes and peritoneal macrophages were harvested and tested in vitro against a ^{51}Chromium bladder tumor target with the addition of PBS, indomethacin (10^{-7}M), mouse leukocyte interferon (500 U/ml), or indomethacin + interferon to parallel samples. Peritoneal macrophages alone expressed slight cytotoxicity, but addition of macrophages to lymphocytes resulted in more consistent increments of cytotoxicity. In vitro indomethacin led to minimal if any enhancement of cytotoxicity. In contrast, interferon markedly enhanced lymphocyte cytotoxicity and slightly enhanced the cytotoxicity of macrophages and lymphocytes together. Indomethacin in vivo led to no substantial increase in either lymphocyte or macrophage cytotoxicity in vitro. Moreover, less cytotoxicity was seen in mixtures of lymphocytes and macrophages from indomethacin-treated animals, and these cytotoxicity levels were not enhanced by indomethacin in vitro. Poly I:C in vivo led to marked stimulation of in vitro lymphocyte cytotoxicity but no further enhancement of cytotoxicity was seen with either in vitro indomethacin or interferon. Inoculation of animals with both indomethacin and poly I:C led to lower levels of enhanced lymphocyte cytotoxicity than was seen after inoculation of poly I:C alone. Macrophage cytotoxicity under these conditions was low and did not add materially to the cytotoxicity seen with splenic lymphocytes. Addition of indomethacin to these samples in vitro led to minimal if any enhancement of cytotoxicity.
{Reproduced from (26) with permission of Academic Press}

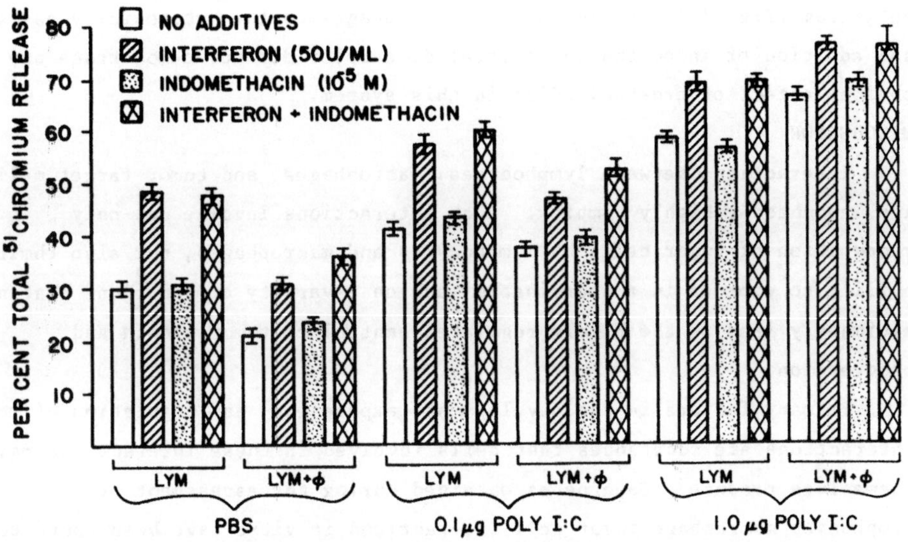

Figure 10. Dose response effect of in vivo poly I:C on lymphocyte (+/- macrophage) cytotoxicity.

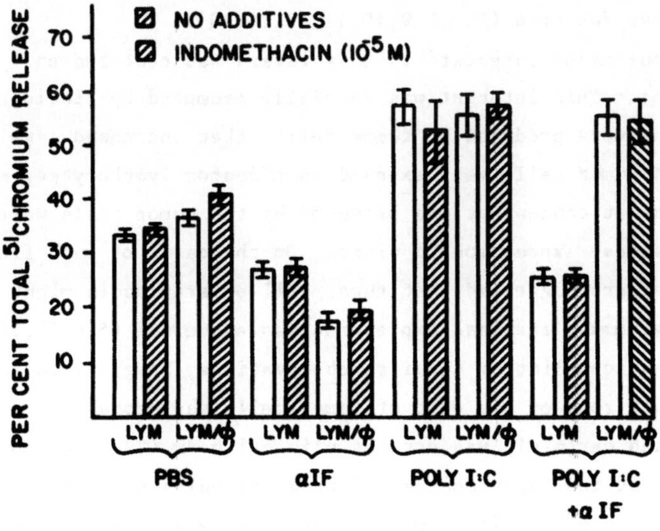

Figure 11. Effect of anti-interferon antiserum (αIF) on poly I:C-enhanced lymphocyte (+/- macrophage) cytotoxicity

cytotoxicity could be prevented by prior inoculation of anti-interferon antiserum (Fig. 11) the presence of macrophages in the cytotoxicity assays, and addition of indomethacin to parallel samples did not demonstrate any obvious effect of prostaglandins in this system.

DISCUSSION

Interactions between lymphocytes, macrophages, and tumor target cells are undoubtedly highly complex. Such interactions involve not only recognition of tumor cells by lymphocytes and macrophages, but also their ability to express in a coordinated fashion a variety of functions that may ultimately lead to the highly regulated control of tumor growth and progression.

Primary factors in the development, expression, and regulation of these interactions are substances that cells involved in these interactions may themselves produce. Supernates obtained during the assessment of lymphocyte/macrophage-tumor cell interactions in vitro have been found to contain a variety of substances with substantial pharmacologic effects on these interactions. These have included promotion or enhancement of the activity of one or another type of cell involved in recognition or effector phases of immune response expression, as well as regulation of the extent of immune response function (2,3,4,9,10,12,13,14,20).

One of our major interests in this regard has centered on prostaglandins. This interest was initially prompted by findings that prostaglandins were produced by tumor cells, that increased levels were produced when tumor cells were exposed to effector lymphocytes, and that prostaglandins at concentrations produced by the tumor cells were inhibitory of immune response expression in vitro. On the basis of such findings, Plescia and others suggested that tumor cell prostaglandin might constitute a means whereby immune response expression was subverted (5,6,15,11). There were sufficient conflicting clinical observations, however, to suggest that a cell regulatory role on the part of tumor cells was probably not generally applicable, and certainly was not the clinical norm (29-32). Moreover, suggestions that the tumor content of prostaglandins was higher than in normal or non-cancerous tissue might also have reflected the presence of macrophages or other host inflammatory cells and their prostaglandin production rather than that of the tumor cells (33).

In vitro prostaglandins had been shown to inhibit lymphocyte mitogenesis, cytolysis, and antibody production in a variety of systems

(34-37). This could be of major importance if the assumptions that an immune response is important in the control of tumor progression, and in primary immune surveillance against tumor development, are correct. Clinical studies in this regard have demonstrated that macrophages from patients with Hodgkin's disease produce excess amounts of prostaglandins; this could be reversed by treatment with indomethacin (38). In patients with breast cancer, prostaglandin synthetase inhibitors caused macrophages in vitro to acquire enhanced cytotoxicity for tumor target cells (39). In patients with head and neck cancers, elevated numbers of prostaglandin inhibitor-sensitive suppressor cells were implicated in a deficient host response to the cancer process (40). Adjuvant administration of indomethacin to these patients led to apparent short-term stabilization of disease.

Our attempts to demonstrate similar phenomena in an in vivo model of bladder cancer were less conclusive. Only slight inhibition of tumor growth was observed with indomethacin, whereas the most pronounced effect characterized those groups that were treated with a combination of biologic response modifiers (polyinosinic:polycytidylic acid, an interferon inducer, plus indomethacin). This suggested that the effect of prostaglandin synthetase inhibition might be largely a passive one, correlating with the concept that prostaglandin production may in large part regulate the ultimate extent of immune response expression. Our attempts to document the effect of indomethacin in this system through in vitro cytotoxicity assays, though suggestive, were inconclusive. Although there is a large body of evidence suggesting that macrophage prostaglandin production may provide a regulatory mechanism for controlling the extent of immune response expression, we were unable to enhance lymphocyte cytotoxicity consistently with indomethacin when macrophages were present during cytotoxicity testing.

Rather than obviating the suggestion that prostaglandins may be important in the control of immune response expression, such results may actually demonstrate the difficulty in projecting observations of in vitro experiments to interpretations of in vivo phenomena. Such projections are complicated further by the likelihood that each cell type involved in such interactions may respond in different ways, at different times, and to different concentrations of the same biologic response modifier. Thus, the timing of exposure and dose of lymphokine in the microenvironment of these cells is probably of critical overall importance in the final expression of activity of each type of cell.

A further indication of this complexity has been suggested in other studies in which prostaglandins were important in the activation of immune response expression as well as the regulation of the extent of this expression. In one study, prostaglandins restored normal host response to interferon, which then enhanced natural cytotoxicity (41,42), while indomethacin and other inhibitors of prostaglandin synthesis abolished this response. In another study, prostaglandins induced increased anti-tumor activity of resident and elicited macrophages (2). Moreover, activation of such macrophages by lipopolysaccharides could be blocked by indomethacin. On the other hand, some have suggested that activated macrophages may lose their capacity to lyse tumor cells as the result of an accumulation of endogenously produced prostaglandins. Stimulation of the macrophage to an activated state may then alter the sensitivity of these cells to exogenous sources of prostaglandins (2).

The importance of the timing of exposure during such interactions has been suggested in studies in which resident macrophages could be stimulated to produce prostaglandins which in turn would activate these macrophages to become tumoricidal (8). However, further accumulation of prostaglandins would then prevent long-term, uncontrolled expression of antitumor cell activity by these activated cells (8,9). Activated macrophages were then found to be far more sensitive to the inhibitory effects of prostaglandins than were non-activated cells (8). A similar differential response to prostaglandins has been observed in lymphocytes, depending upon their state of activation. Thus, lymphocytes have been found to be far more sensitive to prostaglandins when they have been stimulated by suboptimal rather than optimal doses of mitogen (34,37).

Other factors may also enter into the complexity of these interactions. For example, prostaglandins exert a dose-dependent suppression of both T cell growth factor (TCGF) production and action (20). Because this factor is known to promote the clonal expansion of both helper T cells and cytotoxic T cells, the consequences of prostaglandin suppression of TCGF releaser action, and the extent of such suppression, might be reflected in an inhibition of both humoral and cellular immune responses. Through their production of prostaglandin, macrophages could then provide a delicate balance of stimulatory and inhibitory signals to activated T cells. In addition, prostaglandin E_2 has been shown to activate natural killer cell activity, if the cells are exposed to prostaglandin prior to cytotoxicity testing (13).

In contrast, when natural killer cell/target cell conjugates are exposed to prostaglandins during cytotoxicity testing, natural killer activity is inhibited. Augmentation of natural killer cell activity by prostaglandin E_2 has been thought to occur both through increased killing per se as well as by recruitment of "pre-NK" cells that are already target-bound into the active natural killer pool. Whether this reflects the induction of interferon production by prostaglandin, (42) which might itself serve as a recruitment factor, is unknown. Others have suggested a role for activation of a third helper cell or inhibition of an NK suppressor cell by prostaglandin.

In extrapolating from such suggestions, it is not inconceivable that systemic prostaglandin responses could be provoked in the absence of local production. This would enable isolated circulating effector cells to become activated before encountering appropriate targets. If these activated cells then come into contact with targets in an environment of low prostaglandin concentration, overall in vivo expression of activated natural killer cell activity might occur either through direct capacitation by prostaglandins or by their induction of stimulatory lymphokines. Subsequent increased production of prostaglandins by tumor cells in contact with the effector cells would then lead to higher levels of prostaglandins in the microenvironment of the effector cells at a time when such cells are more susceptible to the inhibitory effects of the prostaglandins. Although clearly hypothetical, these suggestions clearly demonstrate the likely complexity of these interactions.

The ability of cells involved in immune response expression to produce other lymphokines, which themselves may either be stimulatory or inhibitory of selected aspects of immune response expression and which may also be effected by prostaglandins, adds further complexity to these interactions (43,44,45). It is also conceivable that a variety of different prostaglandins may be produced by these cells, and that each may have differential effects on immune response expression. These possibilities also remain to be assessed.

Much remains to be learned about these phenomena. If we can assume that the immune response is at all important in the control of tumor development and progression, the role of prostaglandins, because of their ubiquity and profound effect in a variety of in vitro systems, may be of utmost importance. Further characterization of these interactions in all of their ramifications (including types of prostaglandins, concentrations, and timing of events) is necessary if we are to be able to manipulate them successfully in mounting an immunologically based defense against tumor progression.

REFERENCES

1. Tomar RH, Darrow TL, John PA: Response to and production of prostaglandin by murine thymus, spleen, bone marrow, and lymph node cells. Cell Immunol (60):335, 1981.
2. Snider MW, Fertel RH, Zwilling BS: Prostaglandin regulation of macrophage function: effect of endogenous and exogenous prostaglandins. Cell Immunol (74):234, 1982.
3. Koga Y, Taniguchi K, Kubo C, Nomoto K: Peritoneal adherent cells inhibit the generation of cytotoxic T-lymphocytes with prostaglandin-mediated system. Cell ImmunoL (66):195, 1982.
4. Shimamura T, Hashimoto K, Sasaki S: Feedback suppression of the immune response in vivo. II. Involvement of prostaglandins in the generation of suppressor-inducer B lymphocytes. Cell Immunol (69):192, 1982.
5. Karmali RA: Review: prostaglandins and cancer. Prostaglandins Med (5):11, 1980.
6. Goodwin JS: Prostaglandin E and cancer growth potential for immunotherapy with prostaglandin synthetase inhibitors. IN: Hersh EM, Chirigos MA, Mastrangelo MJ (eds) Progress in Cancer Research and Therapy. Augmenting Agents in Cancer Therapy. Raven Press, New York, 1981, vol. 16, p 393.
7. Owen K, Gomolka D, Droller MJ: Lymphocyte-induced production of prostaglandin E_2 by tumor cells in vitro: requirements for direct contact and lymphocyte viability. Cell Immunol (55):428, 1980.
8. McCarthy ME, Zwilling BS: Differential effects of prostaglandins on the anti-tumor activity of normal and BCG-activated macrophages. Cell Immunol (60):91, 1981.
9. Koren HS, Anderson SJ, Fischer DG, Copeland CS, Jensen PJ: Regulation of human natural killing. I. The role of monocytes, interferon, and prostaglandins. J Immunol (127):2007, 1981.
10. Leung KH, Koren HS: Regulation of human natural killing. II. Protective effect of interferon on NK cells from suppression by PGE_2. J Immunol (129):1742, 1982.
11. Droller MJ, Lindgren JA, Claessen HE, Perlmann P: Production of prostaglandin E_2 by bladder tumor cells in tissue culture and a possible mechanism of lymphocyte inhibition. Cell Immunol (47):261, 1979.
12. Brunda MJ, Herberman RB, Holden HT: Inhibition of murine killer cell activity by prostaglandins. J Immunol (124):2682, 1980.
13. Kendall RA, Tarean S: The dual effect of prostaglandin and ethanol on the natural killer cytolytic process: effector activation and NK cell-target cell conjugate lytic inhibition. J Immunol (125):2770, 1980.
14. Drysdale BE, Shin HS: Activation of macrophages for tumor cell cytotoxicity: identification of indomethacin sensitive and insensitive pathways. J Immunol (127):760, 1981.

15. Plescia OJ, Smith AH, Grimwich K: Subversion of the immune system by tumor cells and the role of prostaglandins. Proc Nat Acad Sci (72):1848, 1975.
16. Heney CS, Bourne HR, Lichtenstein LM: The role of cyclic 3'5' adenosine monophosphate in the specific cytolytic activity of lymphocytes. J Immunol (108):1526, 1972.
17. Strom TB, Deisseroth A, Morganroth J, Carpenter CB, Merrill JP: Alteration of the cytotoxic action of sensitized lymphocytes by cholinergic agents and activators of adenylate cyclase. Proc Nat Acad Sci (69):2995, 1972.
18. Goodwin JS: Prostaglandin and regulation of mitogenesis. Cell Immunol (52):239, 1980.
19. Gordon D, Bray MA, Morley J: Control of lymphokine secretion by prostaglandins. Nature (262):401, 1976.
20. Baker PE, Fahey JV, Munck A: Prostaglandin inhibition of T-cell proliferation is mediated at two levels. Cell Immunol (61):52, 1981.
21. Droller MJ, Schneider MU, Perlmann P: A possible role of prostaglandins in the inhibition of natural and antibody-dependent cell-mediated cytotoxicity against tumor cells. Cell Immunol (39):165,m 1978.
22. Droller MJ, Perlmann P, Schneider MU: Enhancement of natural and antibody-dependent lymphocyte cytotoxicity by drugs which inhibit prostaglandin production by tumor target cells. Cell Immunol (39):154, 1978.
23. Erturk E, Price JM, Morris JE, Cohen S, Leith BS, vonEsch AM, Crovetti AJ: The production of carcinoma of the urinary bladder in rats by feeding N-[4-(5-nitro-2-furyl)-2-thiazolyl] formamide. Cancer Res (27):1998, 1967.
24. Owen K, Gomolka D, Droller MJ: Production of prostaglandin E_2 by tumor cells in vitro. Cancer Res (40):3167, 1980.
25. Droller MJ, Gomolka D: Enhancement of natural cytotoxicity in lymphocytes from animals with carcinogen-induced bladder cancer. J Urol (129):625, 1983.
26. Droller MJ, Gomolka D: Interferon induction and prostaglandin synthetase inhibition in the in vitro and in vivo manipulation of immune response expression in an animal model of bladder cancer. Cell Immunol (72):1, 1982.
27. Droller MJ, Gomolka D: Indomethacin and poly I:C in the inhibition of carcinogen-induced bladder cancer in an experimental animal model. Invest Urol, in press, 1984.
28. Droller MJ, Gomolka D: Inhibition of tumor growth in association with modifiction of in vivo immune response by indomethacin and polyinosinic:polycytidylic acid. Cancer Res (42):5038, 1982.
29. Bennett A, Charlier EM, McDonald AM: Prostaglandins and breast cancer. Lancet (2):624, 1977.
30. Bennett A, Carroll MA, Stamford IF: Prostaglandins and human lung carcinoma. Brit J Cancer (46):888, 1982.
31. Khan O, Hensby CN, Williams G: Prostacyclin in prostatic cancer: a better marker than bone scan or serum acid phosphatase? Brit J Urol (54):26, 1982.
32. Caro JF, Besarab A, Flynn JT: Prostaglandin E and hypercalcemia in breast carcinoma: only a tumor marker? A need for perspective. Amer J Med (66):337, 1979.
33. Tanner NS, Stamford IF, Bennett A: Plasma prostaglandins in mucositis due to radiotherapy and chemotherapy for head and neck cancer. Brit J Cancer (43):767, 1981.

34. Goodwin JS: Prostaglandin regulation of mitogenesis. Cell Immunol (52):239, 1980.
35. Murray JL: Prostaglandin E_2 modulation of human monocyte antibody-dependent cell-mediated cytotoxicity against human red blood cells. Cell Immunol (71):196, 1982.
36. Fischer A, Durandy A, Griscelli C: Role of prostaglandin E_2 in the induction of non-specific T lymphocyte suppressor activity. J Immunol (126):1452, 1981.
37. Goodwin JS, Webb DR: Regulation of the immune response by prostaglandins. Clin Immunol Immunopathol (15):106, 1980.
38. Goodwin JS, Messner RP, Bankhurst AD: Prostaglandin-producing suppressor cells in Hodgkin's Disease. New Engl J Med (297):963, 1977.
39. Cameron DJ, O'Brien P: Relationship of the suppression of macrophage medicated tumor cytotoxicity in conjunction with secretion of prostaglandin from the macrophage of breast cancer patients. Int J Immunopharmacol (4):445, 1982.
40. Panje WR, Maca R: Prostaglandin inhibitor sensitive suppressor cells: a product of survival in advanced head and neck cancer. International Symposium on Prostaglandins and Cancer, Washington, D.C., 1981.
41. Favolli C, Leport P, Jaffe BM, Santoro MG, Simmett T, Gobbo VD, Garaci E: The differential effects of PGE on the immune response in normal and immunosuppressed mice. Cell Immunol (72):351, 1982.
42. Stringfellow DA: Prostaglandin restoration of the interferon response by hypoactive animals. Science (201):376, 1978.
43. Taffet SM, Pace JL, Russell SW: Lymphokine maintains macrophage activation for tumor cell killing by interfering with the negative regulatory effect of prostaglandin E_2. J Immunol (127):121, 1981.
44. Tilden AB, Balch CM: A comparison of prostaglandin E_2 effects on human suppressor cell function and on interleukin 2 function. J Immunol (129):2469, 1982.
45. Wolf M, Droege W: Inhibition of cytotoxic responses by prostaglandin E_2 in the presence of interleukin 2. Cell Immunol (72):286, 1982.

These investigations were supported by Grant Number CA24592, awarded by the National Cancer Institute, Department of Health and Human Services.

Chapter 3

THE ROLE OF PGE_2 IN THE INDUCTION OF SUPPRESSOR CELLS IN HUMANS

A. FISCHER, A. DURANDY, F. LE DEIST, C. GRISCELLI

1. INTRODUCTION

Monocytes and related cells play a key role in regulating the interleukin (IL) cascade leading to T cell proliferation and finally to the immune response. They can either amplify the response by producing IL1 (1) or shut it down, mainly by releasing prostaglandin E_2 (PGE_2) (2,3). It has clearly been demonstrated that monocytes can produce sufficient levels of PGE_2 to inhibit all types of immune responses (4-6). PGE_2 acts primarily through the suppression of IL2 production by T lymphocytes (7,8), but some experimental results also suggest the possible interference of PGE_2 with IL2-dependent proliferation (9). The PGE_2 effect has been shown to be associated with a rise in the cyclic AMP (cAMP) level of T lymphocytes (10), although there is no evidence for a direct role of cAMP in mediating PGE_2 suppressor activity.

Whether PGE_2 acts on every helper T cell (at least on every IL2-producing T cell) or activates suppressor T cells remains a matter of discussion. We have studied the role of PGE_2 in the activation of suppressor T cells assayed on T cell proliferation as well as on in vitro B cell maturation driven by pokeweed mitogen (PWM) in humans. After presenting and discussing data giving indirect and direct evidence for PGE_2-inducible T suppressor cells, we will describe attempts at characterizing these cells and examine possible regulatory mechanisms of the monocyte-dependent suppressor circuit. Finally, we will present clinical situations in which the PGE_2 suppressor circuit is disturbed, as already shown by several authors (11,12).

2. INDIRECT EVIDENCE FOR PGE_2 INDUCTION OF T SUPPRESSOR LYMPHOCYTES

Stobo et al. have shown heterogeneity in the response of human lymphocytes to PGE_2, as proliferation of high density cells was strongly suppressed by PGE_2, whereas low density cell responses were enhanced (13). Goodwin et al. have also given evidence for a differential response of T lymphocytes to PGE_2, as there was a striking rise in the cAMP level of T lymphocytes bearing a receptor for IgG (Tγ) after exposure to PGE_2 as compared to the remaining T cells (14).

As shown in Table 1, an excess of monocytes exerts a PGE_2-dependent (indomethacin and anti-PGE_2 antiserum-sensitive) suppressor activity on fresh, but not on 24 hour-incubated or 2,000 rad-irradiated, mononuclear cells (MNL). This has already been reported by Goodwin et al. (15). The suppression can, however, be restored by the addition of a small number of fresh, unirradiated T cells to 24 hour-incubated MNL used as a target for the suppression. A similar effect was observed when the test system was phytohemagglutinin (PHA)-induced proliferation or PWM-induced immunoglobulin containing cell (ICC) generation. Similar data were seen when an excess of monocytes were replaced by increasing concentrations of PGE_2 (16). These results indicate the requirement for fresh, radiation-sensitive T lymphocytes in the expression of PGE_2 inhibitory activity.

3. DIRECT EVIDENCE FOR PGE_2 INDUCTION OF T SUPPRESSOR LYMPHOCYTES

T lymphocytes cultured for 48 h with PGE_2 at a concentration of $\geq 10^{-7}$M and subsequently washed extensively actively suppressed PHA-induced proliferation, mixed leukocyte reaction (MLR) and PWM-induced B cell maturation (Table 2). The effect could also be observed when T lymphocytes without Fcγ receptors were incubated with PGE_2.

That PGE_2 can activate suppressor T lymphocytes has now been shown by a number of groups in various sytems. Webb et al. have shown that PGE_2 activates spleen suppressor T cells from

Table 1. Effect of preincubation or irradiation on PGE_2-dependent monocyte suppressor activity.

	Treatment of cells	PHA-induced proliferation (cpm)	PWM-induced ICC generation ($ICC \times 10^{-3}$)
Fresh MNL	...	42,100 ±11,700	3.5 ±4.6
Fresh MNL	indomethacin (5×10^{-7}M)	98,600 ±18,400	42.1 ±9.4
Fresh MNL	anti-PGE_2 antiserum	114,500 ±24,000	39.5 ±5.1
Fresh MNL	anti-TxB_2 antiserum	44,500 ±15,100	6.8 ±1.9
Irradiated* T + B ratio (4:1)§	0	ND#	28.1 ±6.8
Irradiated T + fresh T + B ratio (2:2:1)	0	ND	7.5 ±8.4
preincubated¶ MNL + fresh T ratio (4:1)	0	51,300 ±17,200	ND
preincubated MNL + irradiated T ratio (4:1)	0	95,600 ±19,000	ND

Results are the means of five experiments ±1 SD. Two x 10^5 MNL or purified cells were added to 1 x 10^5 adherent cells and cultured for 3 d (PHA) or 7 d (PWM). ICC were counted by indirect immunofluorescence using fluorochrome-labelled specific anti-heavychain antisera. [Adapted from (16).]

*Irradiated = 2,000 rad-irradiated.

§Ratio = cell to cell ratio.

#ND = not done.

¶Preincubated = 24 h-preincubated.

Table 2. Generation of T suppressor lymphocyte activity by PGE_2 (percent inhibition).

Treatment of T lymphocytes	PHA-induced lymphocyte proliferation	MLR	PWM-induced ICC
PGE_2 10^{-9}M	0	0	0
PGE_2 10^{-8}M	11.7 ± 9.3	15.2 ± 12.4	0
PGE_2 10^{-7}M	60.2 ± 17.5	69.2 ± 14.6	88.7 ± 17.1
PGE_2 10^{-5}M	66.5 ± 21.3	71.4 ± 17.3	75.0 ± 18.9
0 (24 h) then PGE_2 10^{-5}M	9.9 ± 11.9	9.5 ± 8.0	13.7 ± 10.8
Con A	29.5 ± 11.0	81.3 ± 11.5	79.0 ± 18.6
0 (24 h) then Con A	0	4.4 ± 7.0	13.7 ± 10.3

[Reprinted from (16) with permission of J Immunol.]

the mouse (17). These cells produce peptides which, in turn, suppress the response of T cells (18,19). It must be stressed, however, that this effect was seen only with supraphysiological concentrations of PGE_2 (10^{-5}M) and that our results were obtained with 10-fold higher than physiological concentrations of PGE_2 (10^{-7}M). However, the role of PGE_2 in the activation of suppressor T cells has been indicated by the data from Delfraissy et al. suggesting that the in vitro production of antibodies to TNP by lymphocytes from aged people is suppressed by a PGE_2-activated T suppressor subset (20). Goodwin's group has suggested that PGE_2 at a physiological concentration can activate Tγ suppressor cells (21). Moreover, Chouaib et al. have indicated that a radiosensitive, PGE_2-inducible T suppressor population can suppress the production of IL2 in humans (22). Finally, Rogers et al. have shown that staphylococcal enterotoxin B activates Lyt 2(+) T suppressor cells in a prostaglandin-dependent mechanism (23).

Although these data strongly suggest the induction by PGE_2 of suppressor T cells, they do not demonstrate convincingly that PGE_2 alone, within the physiological range, has such an effect. This will be further discussed later in this chapter.

4. CHARACTERIZATION OF IN VITRO PGE_2-INDUCIBLE T SUPPRESSOR CELLS

Previous results have given evidence that in vitro PGE_2-inducible T suppressor cells are sensitive to preincubation and 2,000 rad irradiation and can (16) or cannot bear (21) Fcγ receptors. Chaouaib and Fradelizi have proposed that both T4(+) and T8(+) cells can be the precursors in humans of PGE_2-inducible T suppressor cells but that only PGE_2-inducible T8(+) cells suppress IL2 production (24).

In an effort to better characterize these cells, we have attempted to isolate T cells that bind PGE_2 from human blood. Several years ago, Melmon et al. showed that some human blood lymphocytes have an affinity for insolubilized PGE_2 (25). Moreover, Goodwin et al. were able to label lymphocytes with tritiated PGE_2 (26), although the presence of specific receptor sites for PGE_2 has not been clearly established. We have studied the possible affinity of blood human T cells for PGE_2 insolubilized on Sepharose 4B beads coated with albumin and used this technique to separate T cells with an affinity for PGE_2. The beads were prepared in the following way (see Reference 27 for a detailed description): BrCN-activated Sepharose 4B or 6-MB beads were coupled to bovine serum albumin. After several washings, PGE_2 (or 6-k$PGF_1\alpha$) was covalently bound to Sepharose 4B or 6-MB albumin according to the method of Melmon et al. (25) using carbodiimide. Fifty to 70% of 10 mg of PGE_2 added were bound to 1 g of beads as measured by a tracer dose of ^{3}H-PGE_2. T lymphocytes separated by rosetting with neuraminidase-treated sheep erythrocytes were incubated with the beads for 30 mn at 37° C in a serumless medium. Binding of T lymphocytes to the beads was monitored microscopically. After the collection of non-binding cells, the cells with an affinity for PGE_2 (or 6-k$PGF_1\alpha$) were detached by adding media containing 20% (v/v) of human serum and by gently shaking the beads. As indicated in Table 3, around 20% of blood T cells bound to the beads and could be further detached, whereas virtually no cells bound albumin alone and only a small percentage bound 6-k$PGF_1\alpha$. The T cells' phenotypes (T4 or T8) of the "PGE_2(+) separated T cells" did not differ significantly from unseparated T lymphocytes [91% T3(+), 41% T4(+) and 33% T8(+) for PGE_2(+) cells versus 90%, 52% and 25.5%, respectively, for PGE_2(-) cells and 90%, 52.5% and 26.5%, respectively, for total T cells].

Table 3. Separation of T cells on SA-PGE_2, SA-6k$PGF_1\alpha$ or SA beads.

Experiment	Recovery* (%)	Percent of eluted cells among total recovered cells from:		
		SA-PGE_2 beads	SA6-k$PGF_1\alpha$ beads	SA beads
1	82	22	7	2
2	48	19	9	1
3	60	32	5	2
4	60	12	...	...
5	60	18	...	...
Mean	64 ± 19.2	20.6 ± 7.3	7 ± 2	1.6 ± 1.6

*Recovery from input cells on SA-PGE_2 beads.

As indicated in Table 4, PGE_2(+) T cells behaved in a significantly different way as compared to unseparated T or PGE_2(-) T cells in proliferation assays. Even when supplemented with a small number of monocytes, they responded poorly to mitogens or antigens. On the other hand, PGE_2(-) T cells responded well and sometimes better than unseparated T cells (data not shown).

Table 4. Mitogen (3 d) or antigen (6 d)-induced cell proliferation of unseparated PGE_2(-) or PGE_2(+) cells.

Cell populations	Lymphocyte proliferation induced by:		
	PHA (cpm)	Candida antigens (cpm)	Tetanus toxoid (cpm)
E(+)	42,500 ± 6,700	15,400 ±2,400	10,600 ±2,600
E(+) (+ PGE_2)	8,700 ±1,200	2,400 ± 500	2,200 ± 300
PGE_2(-)	29,000 ± 4,900	12,700 ±2,000	9,700 ±1,700
PGE_2(-) (+ PGE_2)	26,500 ± 5,500	13,200 ± 2,600	8,800 ±1,500
PGE_2(+)	12,300 ± 4,100	2,600 ± 800	1,900 ± 400

(+ PGE_2) signifies that 10^{-5}M PGE_2 was added to the cells in the culture. Results are the means ± 1 SD of five experiments. Five percent of 4,000 rad-irradiated autologous E(-) cells were added as a source of monocytes. Unstimulated ^{3}HT uptake ranged between 250 and 550 cpm for 3-day cultures and between 200 and 480 for 6-day cultures.

More important, PGE_2(+) T cells actively suppressed T cell proliferation (Tables 5 and 6) and PWM-induced B cell maturation (Table 7), whereas T cells isolated by binding 6-k$PGF_{1\alpha}$ were not suppressive. The suppressive activity was not due to a carryover of PGE_2, since: a) PGE_2(-) cells to which PGE_2 (10^{-5}M) was added, which were then washed, were not suppressive (Table 5, line 5) and b) addition of a high concentration of anti-PGE_2 antiserum to PGE_2(+) T cells did not abrogate their suppressive activity (Table 5, line 7). The suppressor effect was strong, since suppression in a magnitude of 80 to 100% was achieved, and the number of activated suppressor T cells was elevated, since sizeable suppression was observed when 25,000 PGE_2(+) T cells were added to 1 x 10^5 target cells in an

Table 5. Suppressor activity of E(+), PGE_2(-) and PGE_2(+) cells on PHA and allogeneic cell-induced lymphocyte proliferation.

Cells added	PHA (cpm)	MLR (cpm)
0	56,000 ± 7,800	39,300 ± 8,500
E+	57,500 ±6,100	44,900 ±4,000
E(+) (Con A)	20,500 [64] ±4,400	9,200 [79] ±2,700
PGE_2(-)	78,400 [0] ±12,300	39,500 [13] ±4,300
PGE_2(-) (+PGE_2)	70,700 [0] ±14,600	37,200 [18] ±5,200
PGE_2(+)	15,600 [73] ± 1,700	10,500 [77] ± 2,200
PGE_2(+) (+anti-PGE_2 antiserum 1:100)	14,400 [75] ± 1,200	12,500 [72] ± 1,700
6-kPGF$_1\alpha$(-)	68,100 ± 9,400	45,900 [0] ± 6,100
6-kPGF$_1\alpha$(+)	47,900 [17] ±6,200	36,900 [7] ±4,000

Results are the means ± 1 SD of five experiments. The ratio between suppressor cells and responder cells was 1:1. The percentages of suppression are indicated in brackets.

MLR (Table 6). These data indicate that binding of some T lymphocytes to insolubilized PGE_2 led to their activation as nonspecific suppressor T cells. Here, again, the T suppressor cells were activated by highly concentrated, immobilized PGE_2, meaning that isolation of PGE_2(+) cells did not elicit any further information on their physiological role.

It is impossible to determine whether the whole population of PGE_2(+) T cells is suppressive or if it contains other

Table 6. Suppressor activity of E(+), PGE_2(-) and PGE_2(+) cells on allogeneic cell-induced lymphocyte proliferation, depending on the number of suppressor cells added.

Cells added	Suppressor/target ratio				
	0	1:10 (cpm)	1:4 (cpm)	1:2 (cpm)	1:1 (cpm)
E(+)	28,100 ±5,200	30,300 ±8,000	28,500 ±6,200	32,000 ±4,100	35,600 ±5,300
PGE_2(-)		26,700 ±4,800 [12]	32,400 ±7,000 [0]	35,500 ±5,500 [0]	28,000 ±3,700 [21]
PGE_2(+)		27,300 ±5,400 [10]	15,500 ±1,600 [46]	12,600 ±1,100 [61]	7,000 ±1,800 [80]

The number of responder cells was 1 x 10^5, and the number of added suppressor cells is indicated by the ratio (1:10 to 1:1 = suppressor:responder cell). The results are the means ± 1 SD of three experiments. The percentages of suppression are indicated in brackets.

Table 7. Suppressor activity of E(+), PGE_2(-) and PGE_2(+) cells on PWM-induced immunoglobulin containing cell (ICC) generation.

Cells added	Recovered cell number (x 10^{-3})	ICC (x 10^{-3}):		
		IgM	IgG	IgA
0	175 ± 32	22.4 ± 6.8	18.7 ± 7.4	15.4 ± 5.9
E(+)	151 ± 35	20.5 ± 8.7	15.4 ± 5.8	12.3 ± 4.7
PGE_2(-)	138 ± 81	25.3 ± 4.9	19.4 ± 6.5	18.7 ± 5.1
PGE_2(+)	106 ± 52	0.5 ± 0.4	0.3 ± 0.2	$<$0.1

Results are the means ± 1 SD of seven experiments. The ratio between suppressor cells and responder cells was 1:1.

functionally distinguishable populations. In support of the latter hypothesis, opposite roles for PGE_2 have been demonstrated on T cell subsets as well as on B cell function when tested in PWM-induced activation (28-30). It has been proposed, for example, that some suppressor T lymphocytes can be blocked by PGE_2 (28,30). The effect observed with the PGE_2(+) T cell subset may represent, therefore, the addition of opposite actions. Further experiments designed to separate T4(+) PGE_2(+) and T8(+) PGE_2(+) lymphocytes or to use other cell membrane markers are needed to delineate various T cell subsets which have an affinity for PGE_2 but are programmed to different functions. It is likely that PGE_2(+) T cells can also exert other functions, such as the production of osteoclasting activating factor, which is known to be dependent on monocyte PGE_2 (31).

We have described PGE_2(+) T cells as a T cell subset. One cannot, however, rule out the possibility that a larger number of T cells could express PGE_2 receptors, depending upon their state of activation or their cycle phase. Accordingly, one can mention that PGE_2(+) T cells cannot bind PGE_2 again for at least 24 h following separation (data not shown). Modulation of the affinity of T cells for PGE_2 has thus to be studied.

4.1. Role of PGE_2 in the activation of suppressor T cells by Concanavalin A (Con A)

Incubation of T lymphocytes with Con A results in the generation of a suppressor effect that has been shown to be extremely heterogeneous in terms of both the suppressor T cell characteristics and their suppressor mechanisms (32-35). It has been suggested that Con A-activated T cells are suppressive by consuming the IL2 present in the culture or, alternatively, that they are suppressive by secreting partially characterized suppressor factors (34,35). These discrepancies could be due to subtle variations in culture condition. Similar differences have been found when examining the role of PGE_2 in Con A-induced suppression, since Goodwin et al. found that indomethacin enhances Con A-induced T cell suppressor activity (36) in contrast to our own data (Table 8) showing that either indomethacin or an anti-PGE_2 antiserum (but not an anti-TxB_2 antiserum) abrogates the induction of Con A suppressor T cells. It is especially interesting, however, to observe that small concentrations of PGE_2 (10^{-9}M) are required to activate suppressor T cells by Con A. Indeed, incubation in a first step of T cells with Con A and an anti-PGE_2 antiserum followed by the addition 24 h later of 10^{-9}M PGE_2 resulted in the activation of T suppressor

Table 8. Modulation of Con A-induced T suppressor lymphocyte activity.

Treatment of T lymphocytes	Substances added to culture medium	Suppressive effect on MLR (%)	Suppressive effect on PWM-induced ICC generation (%)	N
Con A	...	81.3 ±11.5	79.0 ±18.6	10
Con A + anti-PGE_2 antiserum	...	4.3 ±4.5	12.0 ±20.8	5
Con A + anti-TXB_2 antiserum	...	62.5 ±17.4	98.7 ± 2.4	5
Con A + indomethacin (5×10^{-7}M)	...	21.2 ±11.5	18.5 ±15.2	3
Con A	anti-PGE_2 antiserum	71.2 ± 4.7	77.0 ±11.5	3
Con A + anti-PGE_2 antiserum, then PGE_2 10^{-9}M	...	64.1 ± 15.2	ND	3
Con A + anti-PGE_2 antiserum, then PGE_2 10^{-8}M	...	68.5 ± 12.7	ND	3

[Adapted from (16) with permission of J Immunol.]

cells (Table 8). Although the system used has no in vivo relevance and is controversial, this was the first indication of the role of a physiological dose of PGE_2 in T suppressor activation and was followed by the data of Goodwin et al. (21) concerning the role of PGE_2 in the activation of suppressor Tγ cells. When PGE_2(-) cells isolated as non-binding to PGE_2-coated beads were incubated for 48 h with Con A and then tested for their suppressive activity on MLR or PWM-driven B cell maturation, the various experiments yielded contradictory results, apparently reflecting the complexity of Con A-inducible suppression (Table 9). In four out of six experiments, no suppressor effect was observed on MLR, nor was any observed in four out of four experiments on PWM-driven B cell maturation. In contrast, in two out of six experiments, suppression of MLR

Table 9. Suppression exerted by Con A-activated PGE_2(-) T cells.

Experiment	Suppression (%) exerted on:	
	MLR	PWM-induced ICC
1	0	0
2	0	0
3	0	ND
4	0	ND
5	61	0
6	54	0

Cells were incubated for 48 h with Con A (40 μg/ml) at 37° C, then washed with alphamethylmannoside. Ratio between suppressor and target was 1:1. Suppression is expressed as

$$\left(1 - \frac{\text{cpm or ICC in test culture}}{\text{cpm or ICC in control culture}} \right) \times 100\%.$$

Control culture was performed by adding unseparated T cells or PGE_2(-) T cells similarly cultured for 48 h without Con A.

occurred even when no suppression of B cell maturation was observed. One can speculate that in both experiments in which PGE_2(-) Con A-activated T cells suppressed MLR but not B cell maturation, consumption of IL2 was responsible for the suppression. If this testable hypothesis is correct, it may confirm that PGE_2 at low dose is required for Con A generation of T suppressor cells. Thus, PGE_2, while unable alone to induce T suppressor cells, might at a low physiological dose be a signal for T suppressor activation. In vitro Con A might represent the equivalent of an unknown, putative second signal.

It will be of interest to compare the PGE_2-inducible T suppressor subset with that activable by histamine (37), especially since histamine-induced suppression has been shown to be PGE_2-dependent (38). Moreover, a better evaluation of the role of T suppressor cells with an affinity for PGE_2 requires an adequate assay system for antigen-specific induction of suppressor T cells. Table 10 summarizes the major data concerning the PGE_2(+) T suppressor "subset."

Table 10. Characteristics of the T cell "subset" with an affinity for PGE_2 and with suppressive activity.

- 10 to 30% of human blood T cells
- sensitive to incubation
- radiosensitive (2,000 rads)
- both T4(+) and T8(+) or only T8(+)
- Dr(-)
- contains the Con A-inducible T suppressor subset (?)

5. BACK REGULATION OF PGE_2-DEPENDENT MONOCYTE SUPPRESSOR ACTIVITY

Several groups have demonstrated the presence in human cord blood and maternal blood of suppressor T cells active on PWM-induced B cell maturation (39,40). In contrast, newborn as well as maternal monocytes have been shown to be poorly suppressive both of T cell proliferation and of B cell maturation (41,42) and to secrete low concentrations of PGE_2. Secretion of PGE_2 and suppressor activity of monocytes can be induced in both cases by incubation with zymosan, MLR supernatants or Con A, suggesting a regulatory mechanism (41-43). We thus envisaged that newborn T suppressor cells, or perhaps Con A-activated adult T cells, could down-regulate PGE_2-dependent monocyte suppressor activity. As depicted in Table 11, preliminary data suggest that adult monocytes preincubated with either newborn maternal T lymphocytes or Con A-activated adult T lymphocytes lost the major part of their suppressive activity as assayed

Table 11. Effects of T cell populations on the expression of suppressor activity exerted by monocytes.

Source of T lymphocytes added to monocytes	Pretreatment of T lymphocytes	PHA-induced lymphocyte proliferation	PWM-induced ICC generation
		(% suppression)	
<u>Adult monocytes</u>			
...	...	60	69
Adult T	Con A	15	12
Adult T	...	65	72
Newborn T	...	11	21
<u>Newborn monocytes</u>			
...	...	23	7
Newborn T	...	17	11
Adult T	...	49	62
Adult T	Con A	15	ND
Adult T + anti-PGE_2*	...	8	8

T lymphocytes were added for 24 h at 37° C to T cell-depleted populations at a ratio 10:3. Adherent cells (10^5/well) were then isolated by layering an adequate number of the cell mixture. Two x 10^5 MNL were added and tested for PHA-induced proliferation and PWM-induced B cell maturation. Results are the means of four experiments. [Adapted from (41) and (42).]

*Anti-PGE_2 antiserum was added during both the incubation phase and the suppressive test culture.

on PHA-induced proliferation or PWM-induced B cell maturation. Moreover, newborn monocytes preincubated with Con A-stimulated adult T lymphocytes did acquire a significant suppressive activity that was abrogated by the addition of an anti-PGE_2 antiserum. These results must be extended to PGE_2-activated T suppressor cells in order to evaluate a possible direct feedback mechanism between monocytes and T suppressor cells. It could well be that soluble mediators produced by Con A-stimulated T cells exert a similar regulatory effect on PGE_2-dependent monocyte suppressor activity.

Based on several studies (16,17,18,21,22,27,30,41,43), we have proposed a minimal model for the PGE_2 immunoregulatory circuit (Figure 1). Under various physiological stimuli, monocytes can produce sufficient amounts of PGE_2 to activate T suppressor "a" cells, provided there is a second signal. These cells can shut off IL2 production and helper activityto B cells. According to Ceuppens and Goodwin studies, however, there should be a second T suppressor subset "b" that is down-regulated by PGE_2 (28,30). T suppressor "a" cells or an equivalent can control monocyte suppressor activity, realizing a feedback mechanism. The model contains doubtful points, discussed in this chapter, that need further work either to be established or disproven.

6. CHANGES IN PGE_2-DEPENDENT IMMUNOREGULATION IN DISEASES

At least four types of disturbances in PGE_2-dependent immunoregulation can be found in diseases: a) Excessive PGE_2 production secondary to abnormal monocyte activation or activation of other PGE_2-producing cells, b) low PGE_2 production, c) lack of sensitivity to PGE_2 effect, and d) excessive sensitivity to PGE_2 effect.

6.1. Excessive PGE_2 production

Excessive PGE_2 production has now been shown in several diseases, including chronic infections, especially by microorganisms that are obligate or facultative parasites of macrophages,

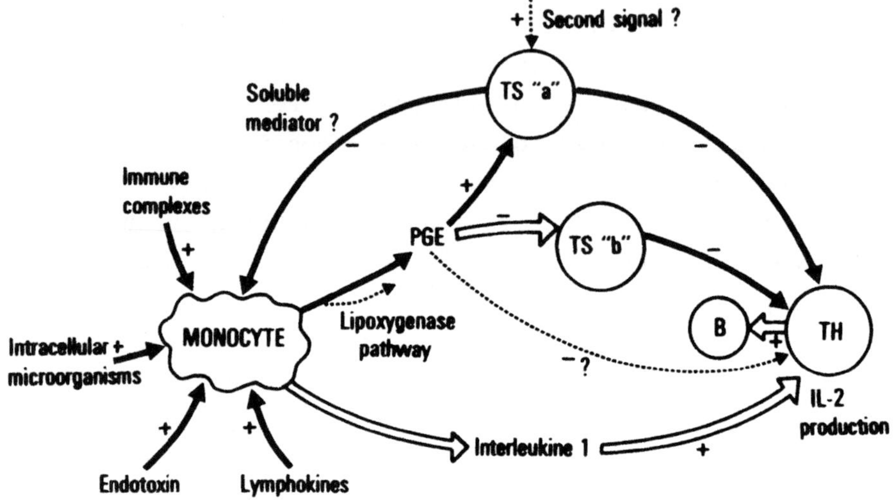

indicates activation

indicates suppression

(as a net balance for the immune response)

FIGURE 1. Working model for the PGE_2 regulatory circuit.

such as mycobacterial infections (44), Chagas disease (45), filariasis (46), coccidiomycosis (47) and cytomegalovirus (CMV) infection (48). We have observed similar excessive PGE_2 production by monocytes together with increased monocyte and T lymphocyte-mediated suppression in infants with congenital rubella (Table 12). Excessive PGE_2 production may at least partially explain the immune deficiency secondary to CMV infection (49).

PGE_2-mediated immunosuppression has been documented in several experimental and human cancers (11,50,51), as detailed in another chapter of this book.

We have extended the study of the immunosuppressive role of PGE_2 to the situation of children without detectable immunodeficiency treated by intramuscular immunoglobulin for upper

Table 12. PGE_2-mediated immunoregulation in congenital rubella.

	Patient 1	Patient 2	Age-matched control
Monocyte PGE_2 production (5 x 10^5 cells/24 h)	15,600	24,300	1,000 - 8,000
Monocyte suppressive activity without indomethacin*	75	81	25
Monocyte suppressive activity with indomethacin*	19	17	20
T suppressive activity exerted on PHA-induced proliferation*	85	90	0

PGE_2 production was evaluated by a radioimmunoassay. The monocyte suppressor activity was evaluated by adding 2 x 10^5 target MNL to 1 x 10^5 adherent cells in a PHA-induced proliferative assay. T cell-mediated suppression was tested at a ratio suppressor/target = 1:1.
*Percent suppression.

respiratory tract infections in whom we found no in vitro response of B cells to PWM (52). As shown in Table 13, we observed the presence of T suppressor cells without prior activation. It was possible to reproduce the phenomenon in vitro by incubating T cells (with 2 to 5% monocytes) with the Ig preparation (but not the fab fragment) that led to T suppressor cell activation. This activation could be blocked by an anti-PGE_2 antiserum. These results are in accordance with the known role of Fc fragments or immune complexes in the induction of PGE_2 secretion by monocytes (53).

Finally, in chronic graft versus host reaction (GVH) following HLA-matched bone marrow transplantation, severe immune deficiency of both cellular and humoral functions was observed together with the presence of non-specific T suppressor cells (54). In three patients with this condition, we also found excessive PGE_2-dependent monocyte suppressor activity and enhanced monocyte PGE_2 production (55) (Table 14) that

Table 13. Suppressor effects of T lymphocytes from patients treated with immunoglobulins or incubated with Ig preparation.

Suppressor population	Number of experiments	ICC IgM	x IgG	10^{-3} IgA
T control	25	8.9	7.8	8.0
T patient	7	.3	.2	.3
T control + Ig	18	.8	.7	1.0
T control + Ig + anti-PGE_2	7	7.6	5.8	6.3
T control + Ig + anti-TxB_2	4	.5	.3	.4

In incubation experiments, T cells (E+) were cultured with Ig preparation (1 mg/ml) for 48 h. T cells were added at a ratio 1:1 to control MNL. [Modified from (52).]

resolved after disappearance of the chronic GVH. It is worth considering that excessive PGE_2 production has been shown in experimental GVH (56) and that PGE_2 production is enhanced by an allogeneic conflict (57). One can thus speculate that PGE_2 plays a role in the immunosuppression observed in chronic GVH.

6.2. Lack of PGE_2 Production

In a unique patient suffering from biotin-dependent multicarboxylase deficiency leading to a defect in fatty acid elongation, among other metabolic abnormalities, we found low PGE_2 production together with low monocyte suppressor activity. The patient's T lymphocytes were not inducible by Con A to suppress, whereas PGE_2 was efficient (58). After in vivo biotin administration, the defect disappeared entirely.

6.3. Lack of Sensitivity to PGE_2

Subjects with the HLA-B12 specificity, as well as patients with multiple sclerosis, have been shown to be less sensitive to the PGE_2 suppressor effect (56,60). In a rare disease, familial erythrophagocytic lymphohistiocytosis, which is characterized by

Table 14. PGE_2-dependent suppression in patients with chronic GVH.

	Patients: 1	2	3	Age-matched control
Monocyte suppressive activity alone*	78	68	77	10-30
Monocyte suppressive activity with indomethacin (5×10^{-7}M)*	18	16	12	5-10
Monocyte suppressive activity with anti-PGE_2*	22	ND	16	5-10
T suppressive activity on PHA-induced proliferation*	90	85	100	0
T suppressive activity on PWM-induced ICC*	95	ND	100	0
PGE_2 pg/ml (5×10^5 adherent cells 1 ml/24 h)	85,000	120,500	45,200	2,000 to 15,000

Two x 10^5 MNL were added to 1 x 10^5 adherent cells and assayed for PHA-induced proliferation. T and B-mediated suppression was evaluated at a ratio suppressor/target = 1:1 for PHA-induced proliferation and PWM-induced B cell maturation.
*Percent suppression.

visceral infiltration by activated macrophages (61), we observed excessive PGE_2 production by monocytes, whereas the patient's T lymphocyte proliferation was not suppressed by his own monocytes. Addition of a small number of control lymphocytes resulted in normal suppression (62). It is possible that a defect of unknown origin in PGE_2-sensitive T suppressor cells resulted in uncontrolled PGE_2 production by monocytes which were thus not normally regulated.

Finally, excessive sensitivity during old age to the immunosupressive effect of PGE_2 has been demonstrated. This has been attributed to suppressor T cells activated by PGE_2 (20).

At least two kinds of data do not fit well with the proposed model (Figure 1). The first is the frequent occurrence of polyclonal hypergammaglobulinemia in patients with excessive PGE_2 production associated with chronic infections or sarcoidosis (63,64). Ceuppens suggests that this is secondary to the blockade by PGE_2 of a T suppressor subset active on helper T cells in polyclonal immunoglobulin production (30). This hypothesis is supported by in vivo data obtained using cyclooxygenase inhibitors (65). However, one cannot rule out the production by monocytes of other mediators, such as IL1, that enhance B cell function (66). Similarly, the excessive PGE_2 production observed in the synovial fluid of patients with rheumatoid arthritis is associated with hypergammaglobulinemia and rheumatoid factor secretion (65).

Although clinical situations point to the possible role of PGE_2-dependent immunosuppression, we are still far from an exact evaluation of this particular immunoregulatory circuit.

REFERENCES

1. Mizel SB: Interleukin 1 and T cell activation. Immunol Rev (63):51-72, 1982.
2. Goodwin JS, Bankhurst A, Messner RP: Suppression of human T-cell mitogenesis by prostaglandin. Existence of a prostaglandin producing suppressor cell. J Exp Med (146):1719-1734, 1977.
3. Kurland JI, Bockman R: Prostaglandin E production by human blood monocytes and mouse peritoneal macrophages. J Exp Med (147):952-957, 1978.
4. Goodwin JS, Webb DR: Regulation of the immune response by prostaglandins. Clin Immunol Immunopathol (15):106-122, 1980.
5. Wolf M, Droege W: Inhibition of cytotoxic responses by prostaglandin E_2 in the presence of interleukin 2. Cell Immunol (72):286-294, 1982.
6. Kurland JI, Kincade PW, Moore MAS: Regulation of B lymphocyte clonal proliferation by stimulatory and inhibitory macrophage-derived factors. J Exp Med (146):1420-1427, 1977.
7. Rappaport RS, Dodge GR: Prostaglandin E inhibits the production of human interleukin 2. J Exp Med (155):943-948, 1982.
8. Walker C, Kristensen F, Bettens F, deWeck AL: Lymphokine regulation of activated (G1) lymphocytes. I. Prostaglandin E2-induced inhibition of interleukin 2 production. J Immunol (130):1770-1773, 1983.

9. Baker PE, Fahey JV, Munik A: Prostaglandin inhibition of T cell proliferation is mediated at two levels. Cell Immunol (61):52-61, 1981.
10. Scott RE: Effects of prostaglandins, epinephrine and NaF on human leukocyte, platelet and liver adenylcyclase. Blood (35):514-521, 1970.
11. Goodwin JS, Messner RP, Bankhurst AD, Peake GT, Saiki JH, Wiliams RC Jr: Prostaglandin-producing suppressor cells in Hodgkin's disease. N Engl J Med (197):263-269, 1977.
12. Plescia OJ, Smith AH, Grinwich K: Subversion of the immune response by tumor cells and the role of prostaglandins. Proc Natl Acad Sci USA (72):1848-1851, 1975.
13. Stobo JD, Kennedy MS, Goldyne ME: Prostaglandin E modulation of the mitogenic response of human T cells. Differential response of T-cell subpopulations. J Clin Invest (64): 1188-1203, 1979.
14. Goodwin JS, Kaszubowski PA, Williams RC Jr: Cyclic adenosine monophosphate response to prostaglandin E_2 in subpopulations of human lymphocytes. J Exp Med (150):1260-1267, 1979.
15. Goodwin JS, Messner RP, Peake GT: Prostaglandin suppression of mitogen-stimulated lymphocytes in vitro. J Clin Invest (62):753-760, 1978.
16. Fischer A, Durandy A, Griscelli C: Role of prostaglandin E_2 in the induction of nonspecific T lymphocyte suppressor activity. J Immunol (126):1452-1455, 1981.
17. Webb DR, Nowowiejski I: Mitogen induced changes in lymphocyte prostaglandin levels: a signal for the induction of suppressor cell activity. Cell Immunol (41):72-78, 1978.
18. Rogers TJ, Nowowiejski I, Webb DR: Partial characterization of a prostaglandin-induced suppressor factor. Cell Immunol (50):82-89, 1980.
19. Rogers TJ, Campbell L, Calhoon K, Nowowiejski I, Webb DR: Suppression of B-cell and T-cell responses by the prostaglandin induced T cell derived suppressor (PITS). Cell Immunol (66):269-276, 1982.
20. Delfraissy JF, Galanaud P, Wallon C, Balavoine JF, Dormont J: Abolished in vitro antibody response in elderly: exclusive involvement of prostaglandin-induced T suppressor cells. Clin Immunol Immunopathol (24):377-385, 1982.
21. Kaszubowski P, Goodwin JS: Monocyte-produced prostaglandin induces Fc gamma receptor expression in human T cells. Cell Immunol (68):343-349, 1982.
22. Chouaib S, Fradelizi D: The mechanism of inhibition of human interleukin 2 production. J Immunol (129):2463-2468, 1982.
23. Donnely RP, Rogers TJ: Inhibitors of prostaglandin synthesis block the induction of staphylococcal enterotoxin B-activated T-suppressor cells. Cell Immunol (81):61-70, 1983.
24. Fradelizi D, Chouaib S: Regulation of IL2 production in man. Abstract from the symposium of the French Society of Immunology on Interleukins 1983, p. 12.

25. Melmon KL, Weinstein Y, Shearer GM, Bourne HR, Bauminger S: Separation of specific antibody-forming mouse cells by their adherence to insolubilized endogenous hormones. J Clin Invest (53):22-35, 1974.
26. Goodwin JS, Wiik A, Lewis M, Bankhurst AD, Williams RC Jr: High affinity binding sites for prostaglandin E on human lymphocytes. Cell Immunol (43):150-158, 1979.
27. Fischer A, LeDeist F, Durandy A, Griscelli C: Separation of a population of human T lymphocytes which bind prostaglandin E_2 and exert a suppressor activity. Submitted for publication, 1984.
28. Gaulde N, Goodwin JS: Effects of prostaglandin E_2 and preincubation on lectin-stimulated proliferation of human T cell subsets. Cell Immunol (70):373-380, 1982.
29. Emilie D, Crevon MC, Galanaud P: Prostaglandin E_2 regulation of human specific B cell response: interaction with a monocyte product. Clin Immunol Immunopathol (29):415-423, 1983.
30. Ceuppens J, Goodwin JS: Endogenous prostaglandin E enhances polyclonal immunoglobulin production by tonically inhibiting T suppressor cell activity. Cell Immunol (70):41-54, 1982.
31. Yoneda T, Mundy GR: Monocytes regulate osteoclast activating factor production by releasing prostaglandin. J Exp Med (150):338-351, 1979.
32. Herscowitz HB, Sakane T, Steinberg AD, Green I: Heterogeneity of human suppressor cells induced by concanavalin A as determined in simultaneous assays of immune function. J Immunol (124):1403-1410, 1980.
33. Palacios R, Möller G: T cell growth factor abrogates Con A-induced suppressor cell function. J Exp Med (153):1360-1365, 1981.
34. Greene WC, Fleisher TA, Waldmann TA: Soluble suppressor supernatants elaborated by concanavalin A-activated human mononuclear cells. I. Characterization of a soluble suppressor T cell proliferation. J Immunol (126):1185-1191, 1981.
35. Fleisher TA, Greene WC, Blaese RM, Waldmann TA: Soluble suppressor supernatants elaborated by concanavalin A-activated human mononuclear cells. II. Characterization of a soluble suppressor of B cell immunoglobulin production. J Immunol (126):1192-1197, 1981.
36. Goodwin JS: Modulation of concanavalin A induced suppressor cell activation by prostaglandin E_2. Cell Immunol (49):421-425, 1980.
37. Rocklin RE: Modulation of cellular immune responses in vivo and in vitro by histamine receptor-bearing lymphocytes. J Clin Invest (57):1051-1060, 1976.
38. Beer DJ, Rosenwasser LJ, Dinarello CA, Rocklin R: Cellular interactions in the generation and expression of histamine-induced suppressor activity. Cell Immunol (69):101-112, 1982.
39. Durandy A, Fischer A, Griscelli C: Active suppression of B lymphocyte maturation by two different newborn T lymphocyte subsets. J Immunol (123):2644-2650, 1979.

40. Hayward AR, Lydyard PM: Suppression of B lymphocyte differentiation by newborn T lymphocytes with an Fc receptor for IgM. Clin Exp Immunol (34):374-378, 1978.
41. Fischer A, Durandy A, Mamas S, McCall E, Dray F, Griscelli C: Lack of prostaglandin E2-mediated monocyte suppressive activity in newborn and mothers. Clin Exp Immunol (49): 377-385, 1982.
42. Durandy A, Fischer A, Griscelli C: Inability of newborns or pregnant women's monocytes to suppress pokeweed mitogen-induced responses. J Immunol (128):525-529, 1982.
43. Durandy A, Fischer A, Mamas S, Dray F, Griscelli C: Respective roles and interactions of T-lymphocyte and PGE_2-mediated monocyte suppressive activities in human newborns and mothers at the time of delivery. Am J Reprod Immunol (2):127-134, 1982.
44. Kleinhenz ME, Ellner JJ, Spagnuolo PJ, Daniel TM: Suppression of lymphocyte responses by tuberculous plasma and mycobacterial arabinogalactan. Monocyte dependence and indomethacin reversibility. J Clin Invest (68):153-162, 1981.
45. Kierszenbaum F: Immunologic deficiency during experimental chagas disease (trypanosoma cruzi infection). J Immunol (129):2202-2205, 1982.
46. Piessens WF, Partono F, Hoffman SL, Ratiwayanto S, Piessens PW, Falmieri JR, Koiman I, Dennis DT, Carney WP: Antigen specific suppressor T lymphocytes in human lymphatic filariasis. N Engl J Med (307):144-148, 1982.
47. Catanzaro A: Suppressor cells in coccidiomycosis. Cell Immunol (64):235-245, 1981.
48. Howard RJ, Najarian JS: Cytomegalovirus-induced immune suppression. Clin Exp Immunol (18):109-126, 1974.
49. Rinaldo CR, Carney WP, Richter BS, Black PH, Hirsch MS: Mechanisms of immunosuppression in cytomegaloviral mononucleosis. J Infect Dis (141):488-495, 1980.
50. Kazimiera D, Grinwich KD, Plescia OJ: Tumor mediated immunosuppressor: prevention by inhibitors of prostaglandin synthesis. Prostaglandins (14):1175-1182, 1977.
51. Rolland PH, Martin PM, Jacquemier J, Rolland AM, Toga M: Prostaglandin in human breast cancer: evidence suggesting that an elevated prostaglandin production is a marker of high metastatic potential for neoplastic cells. JNCI (64): 1061-1070, 1980.
52. Durandy A, Fischer A, Griscelli C: Dysfunctions of pokeweed mitogen-stimulated T and B lymphocyte responses induced by gammaglobulin therapy. J Clin Invest (67):867-877, 1981.
53. Passwell J, Dayer JM, Merler E: Increased prostaglandin production by human monocytes after membrane receptor activation. J Immunol (123):115-120, 1979.
54. Tsoi MS: Immunological mechanisms of graft versus host disease in man. Transplantation (33):459-464, 1982.
55. Fischer A, Durandy A, Griscelli C: T lymphocyte and prostaglandin E2-dependent monocyte suppressor activities found in bone marrow transplanted patients. Fifth International Congress of Immunology, Kyoto, 1983.

56. Lapp WS, Mendes M, Kirchner H, Gemsa D: Prostaglandin synthesis by lymphoid tissue of mice experiencing a graft versus host reaction: relationship to immunosuppression. Cell Immunol (50):271-281, 1980.
57. Dy M, Astoin M, Rigaud M, Hamburger J: Prostaglandin (PG) release in the mixed lymphocyte culture; effect of presensitization by a skin allograft; nature of the PG-producing cell. Eur J Immunol (10):121-126, 1980.
58. Fischer A, Munnich A, Saudubray JM, Mamas S, Coude F-X, Charpentier C, Dray F, Frézal F, Griscelli C: Biotin-responsive immunoregulatory dysfunction in multiple carboxylase deficiency. J Clin Immunol (2):35-38, 1982.
59. Staszak CS, Goodwin JS, Troup GM: Decreased sensitivity to prostaglandin and histamine in lymphocytes from normal HLA-B12 individuals: a possible role in auto-immunity. J Immunol (125):181-185, 1980.
60. Goodwin JS, Messner RP: Prostaglandin E inhibition of mitogen stimulation in patients with multiple sclerosis. Prostaglandins (15):281-286, 1978.
61. Ladisch S, Holiman B, Poplack DG, Blaese RM: Immuno-deficiency in familial erythrophagocytic lymphohistiocytosis. Lancet (1):581-614, 1978.
62. Fischer A, Durandy A, Griscelli C, Mamas S: Prostaglandin E2-mediated monocyte suppressive activity--role in immunoregulatory disorders in primary immuno-deficiencies. (Seligmann and Hitzig W, eds) North Holland, Elsevier, 1980, pp. 363-372.
63. Ceuppens JL, Rodriguez M, Goodwin JS: Non steroidal anti-inflammatory agents inhibit the synthesis of IgM rheumatoid factor in vitro. Lancet (1):528-530, 1982.
64. Goodwin JS, Dehoratius R, Israel H, Peake GT, Messner RP: Suppressor cell function in sarcoidosis. Ann Intern Med (90):169-175, 1979.
65. Goodwin JS, Ceuppens JL: Effect of non steroidal anti-inflammatory drugs on immune function. Semin Arthritis Rheum (13):134-143, 1983.
66. Hoffman M: Macrophages and T cells controls distinct phases of B cell differentiation in the humoral immune response in vitro. J Immunol (125):2076-2080, 1980.

ACKNOWLEDGEMENTS

We are grateful to Ms. C. Barbat, M. Chartier and A. M. Alharie for excellent technical assistance and to S. Mamas for prostaglandin dosages.

Chapter 4

THE ROLE OF ARACHIDONIC ACID METABOLITES IN THE FUNCTION OF MURINE SUPPRESSOR CELLS

THOMAS J. ROGERS

1. INTRODUCTION

A great deal of attention has recently been focused on the role of the products of arachidonic acid metabolism in the regulation of the immune response. It has been suggested by numerous investigators, and in a variety of experimental systems, that several arachidonic acid metabolites may alter lymphocyte function. The primary focus of this chapter is a review of the suppressive activities of the products of arachidonic acid metabolism, with particular emphasis on their role in regulatory (suppressor) cell function.

2. THE REGULATION OF LYMPHOCYTE FUNCTION BY LIPOXYGENASE PRODUCTS

Recent evidence reported in the literature suggests that at least some of the lipoxygenase products may have inhibitory effects on lymphocyte activity. Leukotriene D_4 (LTD_4) and LTE_4 have been shown to suppress both phytohemagglutinin (PHA)- and bacterial lipopolysaccharide (LPS)-induced blastogenic responses, as well as anti-sheep erythrocyte (SRBC) antibody responses (1). The blast transformation reactions were found to be significantly suppressed by as little as nanomolar quantities of these leukotrienes. Recent studies have also shown that 15-hydroxyeicosatetraenoic acid (15-HETE) inhibits murine lymphocyte transformation (2). Although 15-hydroperoxyeicosatetraenoic acid (15-HPETE) and LTB_4 have been shown to suppress PHA-induced mitogen responses of human lymphocytes (3,4), it has been reported that both LTC_4 and LTD_4 are not suppressive for human cells (4). It is most likely that products of the lipoxygenase pathway do have some immunomodulatory activity; however, the significance of

J.S. Goodwin (ed.), PROSTAGLANDINS AND IMMUNITY.

these factors in regulating immune responses in vivo remains to be defined.

3. SUPPRESSION OF LYMPHOCYTE FUNCTION BY CYCLOOXYGENASE PRODUCTS

3.1. Suppressor macrophage activity

It has been known for some time that although lymphoproliferative responses are dependent, in general, on minimal macrophage levels, higher macrophage concentrations exhibit inhibitory effects (see 5 for review). Of course it is clear that a wide range of immunomodulatory substances may be secreted by macrophages (e.g., macrophage dialyzable factor [6]; low-molecular-weight suppressor [7]; macrophage soluble material [8]; and macrophage suppressor factor [9]), and several of these substances are significantly suppressive.

Among the better-defined substances with inhibitory activity are prostaglandins E_1 (PGE_1) and E_2. These prostaglandins have been shown by a variety of investigators to possess inhibitory activity in numerous immunological assays. Among these activities is an inhibition of cytotoxic T cell activity (10-15), natural killer cell activity (16-20), antibody-dependent cytotoxic cell activity (16,17,21,22), interleukin-2 production (23-25), migration inhibition factor production (26,27), mixed-lymphocyte reaction-associated proliferation (28), and mitogen-induced blastogenic responses (29-33). Primary antibody responses to the T-dependent antigen SRBC (34-36), and the T-independent antigen polyvinylpyrrolidone (37), are suppressed by PGE. However, secondary antibody responses to SRBC (38,39), bovine serum albumin, human gamma globulin (39), keyhole limpet hemocyanin (40,41), and DNP-ascaris (42) may be enhanced by PGE. The basis for this dichotomy in the effect of PGE on antibody production is still unclear, but may be due to a differential sensitivity of the various lymphocyte populations to the effects of PGE. Some support for this hypothesis does exist in studies on mitogen-induced lymphocyte proliferation (43,44).

Additional support for the suppressive activity of PGE has come from the use of PG synthetase (cyclooxygenase) inhibitors. The use of drugs such as aspirin, indomethacin, or 5,8,11,14-

eicosatetraynoic acid (ETYA) must be viewed with the understanding that other metabolic effects (related and unrelated) have been reported for these compounds (especially at levels above 100 nM). These effects include an inhibition of membrane receptor-ligand binding (45,46), toxicity (47), and an alteration of cyclic AMP phosphodiesterase (48,49), phospholipase (50), protein synthesis (51), and fatty acid peroxidase (52). With this possible caveat in mind, it should be pointed out that experiments with these compounds have almost always been consistent with the results obtained through the use of PGE directly. In this way, a variety of PG synthetase inhibitors have been shown to enhance killer cell activity (16,19), cytotoxic T cell activity (12,13,15), antibody-dependent cellular cytotoxicity (16), mixed-lymphocyte-induced proliferation (53), interleukin-2 production (23), and mitogen-induced blastogenic responses (34,54). The study of the effects of PG synthetase inhibitors on antibody production has not been entirely straightforward. Several investigators have observed enhanced primary antibody responses in the presence of indomethacin (36,37,53), yet Webb and Nowowiejski (36) and Zimecki and Webb (37) have observed that enhancement (or occasionally suppression) due to the drug is dependent on the antigen dose and the basal level of the immune response. Along these same lines, Schleimer and Benjamini (55) have reported an enhanced primary antibody response to SRBC and a reduced response to chicken serum albumin in the presence of indomethacin. It should be pointed out that a suppression in the primary antibody response to SRBC in the presence of indomethacin has been reported by Barasoain et al. (56). These results are consistent with data reported by Wieder and Webb (39) in which secondary antibody responses to SRBC and bovine serum albumin were found to be reduced in the presence of indomethacin. The reasons for the inconsistency in the effects of these drugs on the antibody response remains unclear at this time.

Cyclooxygenase products are secreted in relatively high concentrations by macrophages. Indeed, the macrophage appears to be the predominant source of PGE among cells of the immune system (57,58). The synthesis of measurable quantities of PGE by lymphocytes has also been reported by some (54, 59), but it should be acknowledged that the lymphocyte may not be a source of immunomodulatory levels of these arachidonic acid metabolites.

Consistent with the observed suppressive activities of PG, and the ability of macrophages to secrete these mediators (especially after "activation" [58,60,61]), a number of investigators have described experimental situations in which macrophages exhibit significant suppressive activity. Gemsa (60) has reported that macrophages recovered from *Corynebacterium parvum*-treated mice exhibit a significant elevation in the release of the cyclo-oxygenase products PGE and thromboxane B2 after 4 days. Prostaglandin E levels return to normal by about day 16. The lymphocyte mitogenic response to concanavalin A in these *C. parvum*-treated mice exhibit significant suppression during the same period of time. The suggestion that PGE produced by macrophages might be responsible for the immunosuppression in these studies is supported by the fact that indomethacin or removal of adherent macrophages alleviates the suppression. Similarly, Lapp et al. (62) have shown that mice undergoing a graft-versus-host reaction manifest elevated splenic PGE levels and reduced responses to PHA and LPS. Depletion of macrophages or treatment with indomethacin reduces the PGE levels, and at least partially returns the responses to mitogen to normal. Significant suppressor-macrophage activity, mediated at least in part by the synthesis and secretion of PGE, has also been reported in the human (63), rat (64-66), and other mouse (66,67) systems.

Macrophages are capable of secreting significant levels of other cyclooxygenase products as well as various lipoxygenase products (58,68), and it may become clear at some time that the suppressive activity of macrophages is due to more than the simple synthesis of PGE. In any case, the suppressive activity of macrophages is apparently due primarily to the release of PGE. More work is clearly needed to understand the role of these suppressive macrophages in the regulation of immune responses by lymphoid cells.

3.2. Suppressor lymphocyte activity

3.2.1. Non-antigen-induced suppressor cell function. Experiments first reported by Folch and Waksman (69) demonstrated the presence in rats of an adherent lymphocyte with suppressive activity. These studies were extended to mice in studies by Webb and Jamieson (33) in which glass wool-adherent T cells (GAT) were found to suppress the PHA-induced blastogenic response. Splenocytes depleted of glass-adherent lymphocytes (GAL) were found to manifest much greater responses to PHA than non-fractionated cells. Further, when GAL (or GAT) were co-cultured with non-adherent lymphocytes (NAL), the response of the NAL were significantly suppressed. These suppressor cells were found to be insensitive to treatments with mitomycin C, actinomycin D, or cycloheximide, indicating that DNA and most protein synthesis were not required for the activity of these suppressor cells. Treatment of these cells with indomethacin, d,l-6-chloro-α-methylcarbozole-2-acetic acid (RO-20-5720), or octadeca-9,12,-diynoic acid (RO-3-1314) inhibited the glass-adherent suppressor cell activity (33,54). These experiments provided the first indication that endogenous prostaglandin synthesis is involved in the regulation of lymphocyte function.

The dependence on PG synthesis suggests the possibility that the suppression in the glass wool-adherent cultures is due to the direct effects of these mediators. As would be expected, preparations of GAL, enriched for T cells by treatment with anti-immunoglobulin and complement, were found to synthesize measurable quantities of PG in response to stimulation by PHA (54). Non-adherent cells (which contain 1-5% contaminating macrophages), and NAL passed over Sephadex G-10 to further deplete the macrophage population, also produce measurable PG following stimulation by PHA. Levels of PG (primarily PGE) increase from 0.37 ng per ml before to 2.2 ng per ml after 48 hours of stimulation with PHA. These levels of PG are significantly less than the level produced by GAL, but the net increase in the PG is significantly greater (10-fold versus 2-fold). It is worth noting that these results suggest macrophage-depleted cultures are capable of some synthesis of PG (as has been suggested by others).

It should be pointed out that the response to PHA of the NAL population is not enhanced by indomethacin, even though these cells are capable of generating measurable PG (54). In fact, enhancement of the response to PHA was only observed in cell cultures containing GAT. The results suggest that suppression of the response to PHA is not due to the direct effects of PGE on the responding T cell population. Webb and Nowowiejski (54) have suggested that PG synthesized by both NAL and GAL may be influencing the activity of a suppressor cell population in the GAT preparation. Support for this suggestion was observed in experiments in which GAT manifested suppressive activity after treatment with a PG synthetase inhibitor as long as exogenous PGE is present. These investigators also observed that supernatants obtained from GAT stimulated with exogenous PGE manifested significant suppressive activity. Webb and Nowowiejski suggested a model to explain the function of the GAT suppressor cell in which PHA stimulates PG synthesis in the NAL (and GAL) population which serves, in turn, to induce a population of T-suppressor cells to release a suppressor factor.

More recent studies by Rogers et al. (70) have shown that the PG-induced T cell-derived suppressor factor (PITS) is actually a mixture of at least two factors. The larger factor ($PITS_{\alpha}$) has an apparent molecular weight of 35 kd and the smaller factor ($PITS_{\beta}$) has an apparent molecular weight of 2-5 kd. Both the $PITS_{\alpha}$ and $PITS_{\beta}$ factors are sensitive to treatment with the proteolytic enzymes trypsin (TPCK-treated), carboxypeptidase A, leu-aminopeptidase, clostropain, chymotrypsin, pronase, or proteinase K, but not to RNase or DNase (70,71). Although the results suggest that the PITS factors possess a protein or peptide moiety required for suppressive activity, the $PITS_{\beta}$ factor is not sensitive to treatment by boiling for 10 minutes (70). These factors suppress both LPS- and PHA-induced proliferative responses, and their activity is apparently not restricted at the H-2 locus. Additional studies have shown that the production of these PITS factors is not inhibited by treatment with cycloheximide (70). This result is consistent with the earlier work reported by Webb and Jamieson (33) which demonstrated that the suppressive activity of GAL cultures is not inhibited by treatment with cycloheximide.

Further work (72) has shown that the production of PITS is due to the direct interaction of PGE with the GAT suppressor cell. An increase in intracellular or extracellular cAMP does not induce significant levels of PITS factor. Furthermore, stimulation with $PGF_{2\alpha}$ (even at 10 μM) does not induce significant production of PITS (5.8 units with $PGF_{2\alpha}$ as compared to 39.9 units with PGE_2). It should be noted that in all of these studies a very high level of PGE (10 μM) is employed to induce PITS production. We have found that levels of PGE_2 as low as 0.1 μM are capable of inducing measurable PITS activity from GAT cultures (unpublished results). Because of the greater production of PITS at the higher concentrations of PGE, the 10 μM level is employed for the further analysis of PITS activity.

More recent studies on the biological activity of the $PITS_\beta$ factor have suggested that this material exerts a broad range of suppressive effects. A report by Rogers et al. (73) has shown that both the allogeneic and syngeneic mixed-lymphocyte reactions are suppressed by $PITS_\beta$. Antibody responses to the T-dependent antigen SRBC, as well as the T-independent antigens DNP-ficoll and DNP-polyvinylpyrrolidone, are also suppressed. The proliferative response to PHA, the antibody responses, and the mixed-lymphocyte reaction are all suppressed to a similar extent with identical doses of $PITS_\beta$ factor.

Studies by these investigators have also shown that treatment with $PITS_\beta$ factor for as little as 2 to 4 hours is sufficient for significant suppression to occur. Splenocytes were treated with $PITS_\beta$ for 4 hours, washed to remove free PITS, and then tested to assess the ability to manifest normal responses. These "short-term"-treated cells fail to manifest normal proliferative responses to PHA, normal antibody responses to SRBC or DNP-ficoll, or a normal mixed-lymphocyte reaction. These results are of particular interest in view of the earlier work which had shown that the production of PITS by GAT occurs within the first 4-6 hours of incubation with PGE (72). Taken together, these results suggest that (at least at high levels of PGE) the production of PITS by GAT, as well as the subsequent effect of the PITS on target cells, may all occur within a total of about 8 hours after contact with PGE.

In an effort to further characterize the PITS$_{\beta}$ factor, we have attempted to purify the factor through the use of conventional size-exclusion chromatography followed by high-pressure liquid chromatography (HPLC). We have found that the PITS$_{\beta}$ factor is actually a mixture of at least seven distinct suppressor factors (T.J. Rogers, J. DeHaven, R.P. Donnelly and B. Lamb, submitted for publication). These studies have shown that although each of these factors suppresses the proliferative response to PHA, PITS$_{\beta 3}$ and PITS$_{\beta 4}$ do not suppress the antibody response to SRBC or the mixed-lymphocyte reaction (see Table 1). The conditions of elution (40% propanol in 0.1 M ammonium acetate, pH 5.5) of these factors from this type of column indicate that these factors are moderately hydrophobic.

Table 1. Suppressive activity of the PITS$_{\beta}$ factors.

	Suppressive Activity						
Function	β1	β2	β3	β4	β5	β6	β7
Response to PHA	+	+	+	+	+	+	+
Antibody to SRBC	+	+	-	-	+	+	+
MLR	+	+	-	-	+	+	+

In order to generate large quantities of these factors, we have attempted to create lymphocyte hybridomas which produce any or all of these PITS$_{\beta}$ factors. The T-lymphoma BW-5147 has been used as a fusion partner with C57Bl/6 GAT in the creation of the T cell hybridomas (74,75). We have been successful in isolating two hybridoma clones which appear to constitutively synthesize three of these suppressor factors (T.J. Rogers, J. DeHaven and R.P. Donnelly, submitted for publication). The results show that hybridoma clone Hyb-7SC2 produces factors which co-elute (by HPLC) with the PITS$_{\beta 2}$ and PITS$_{\beta 5}$ factors, while hybridoma clone Hyb-9SC2 produces a factor which co-elutes with PITS$_{\beta 1}$. The parental BW-5147 cell line does not produce measurable PITS$_{\beta}$ activity. As in the case of the conventional PITS$_{\beta 1,2}$ and $_5$ factors, hybridoma-derived factors suppress the proliferative response to PHA, the antibody response to SRBC, and the mixed-lymphocyte reaction. These two clones possess both Thy-1.1 and Thy-1.2 surface antigens, as well as both parental (and intermediate) forms of glucose phosphate isomerase isozymes (74,75), indicating that these clones do indeed express gene products from the C57Bl/6 fusion partner.

Work done in collaboration with D. Webb and his colleagues has provided some insight into the biochemical nature of $PITS_{\beta 6}$ (D.R. Webb, K.J. Wieder, T.J. Rogers, C.T. Healy and I. Nowowiejski-Wieder, submitted for publication). Treatment of GAT cultures with indomethacin together with PGE increases the suppressor factor production, while ETYA (an inhibitor of both the lipoxygenase and cyclooxygenase activities) together with PGE inhibits factor production. In addition, both radiolabeled arachidonic acid and cysteine are incorporated by GAT into the PITS factor. As would be expected for a leukotriene, PITS factor is also active in the guinea pig ileum assay. And finally, $PITS_{\beta 6}$ factor co-elutes (by HPLC) with LTE_4. Taken together, these results suggest that $PITS_{\beta 6}$ is a leukotriene or leukotriene-like molecule. These results are consistent with an earlier report in which we showed that LTD_4 and LTE_4 are both capable of suppressing the proliferative response to PHA as well as the antibody response to SRBC (1). It is not currently thought that lymphocytes are capable of significant leukotriene synthesis, but our results indicate that both LTD_4 and LTE_4 may be active at nanomolar levels (1). Still, the possibility does exist that $PITS_{\beta 6}$ is the product of contaminating non-lymphoid cell types in the GAT preparation.

3.2.2. Mitogen-induced suppressor cell function. The T cell mitogen concanavalin A (Con A) is capable of inducing potent T-suppressor (Ts) cell activity. These cells bear the "typical" cell surface markers Thy-1 and Lyt-2,3, and function in an antigen-nonspecific fashion (76). Recent reports from the laboratory of C. Pierce have suggested that Con A induces the synthesis of a suppressor factor, the soluble immune response suppressor (SIRS), which apparently functions by inducing macrophages to release a second factor (the macrophage-derived suppressor factor, Mϕ-SF) (77,78). The Mϕ-SF is a protein with a molecular weight of

50-55 kd which is released between 24 and 72 hours after a 2-hour exposure to SIRS (78). Antibody responses and both the T cell- and B cell-dependent proliferation in response to mitogens are suppressed by the Mϕ-SF (78). It is not clear at this time whether all Con A-induced Ts cell activity is due to the production of SIRS and Mϕ-SF.

Studies on the role of PG synthesis in the function of these Con A-activated suppressor cells have yielded contradictory results. Studies in three independent laboratories (79-81) on Con A-induced human Ts cells have suggested that inhibition of PG synthesis by indomethacin enhances the suppressive activity. Results reported by Kemp et al. (66), Badger et al. (82), and Leung et al. (83) suggest that Con A-activated murine Ts cells are either not affected, or are enhanced, in the presence of indomethacin. Taken together, these results suggest that PG is not required for Ts cell activity, and that suppressor activity may actually be inhibited by PG. These results are in direct conflict with results reported by Orme and Shand (84,85) for murine cells, and Fischer et al. (86) for human cells, which have suggested that inhibition of PG synthesis results in a reduction in Con A-induced suppressor cell activity. The basis for the disagreement in the literature concerning the effects of indomethacin on Con A-induced Ts cell function remains unclear. It is possible that Con A may activate more than a single population of Ts cells, and under particular experimental conditions, the function of only one or a portion of these populations may be evident. It may be possible, for example, that one or more populations of these cells may function independently of the SIRS/Mϕ-SF system. It is conceivable, therefore, that if one population of Con A-activated Ts cells is dependent on PG synthesis, and the other is not, that contradictory results may be obtained.

We have recently described the activation of Ts cells with the T cell mitogen Staphylococcal enterotoxin B (SEB) (87). These Ts cells bear the Thy-1 and Lyt-2,3 surface markers. Furthermore, both the induction and expression of SEB-induced T-suppressor (SEB-Ts) cells appear to be macrophage independent. Our most recent results (Y.-S. Lin, M. Holly and T.J. Rogers, unpublished observations) suggest that the SEB-Ts cells are distinct, both in terms of the mechanism of induction and expression, from the Con A-induced Ts cells.

We have attempted to assess the role of arachidonic acid metabolism in the induction and expression of the SEB-Ts cells. A report by Donnelly and Rogers (88) has shown that inhibitors of the cyclooxygenase pathway (such as indomethacin and ETYA) block the induction of SEB-Ts cell activity. Agents which block the lipoxygenase pathway or thromboxane synthesis (without inhibiting PG synthesis), such as nordihydroguiaretic acid, imidazole, and pyrogallol, do not have any effect on suppressor cell activity. Futhermore, the requirement for PG synthesis occurs in the first 4-6 hours after stimulation with SEB. Inhibition of PG synthesis at later times in the SEB-induction period has no effect on Ts cell activity. This result suggests that these Ts cells do not suppress by simply producing PG. We have also shown that the requirement for PG synthesis in the first 4-6 hours exists even for macrophage-depleted cultures. We suggest that the Ts cells specifically, or another non-macrophage population in the culture, must synthesize PG in order to yield Ts cell activity.

We have also attempted to overcome the indomethacin effect on Ts cells by elevating levels of cAMP (88). Indomethacin has been shown to reduce basal levels of, as well as antigen-induced elevations in, cAMP in splenocytes (89). Our results show that both theophylline (an agent which inhibits phosphodiesterase) and isoproterenol (an adenyl cyclase activator) have no effect on the abrogation of Ts cell activation by indomethacin. It should be noted that Winchurch et al. (90) have suggested that the induction of suppressor cells by LPS is dependent on an elevation in the level of cAMP. The deviation in the requirements for elevated cAMP by SEB-induced Ts cells and the LPS-induced suppressor cells may reflect the fact that LPS induces suppressor cells which possess characteristics of B lymphocytes (91-93).

4. CONCLUSIONS

It is clear that several arachidonic acid metabolites, especially PGE, are capable of directly inhibiting lymphoid function. Not all immune responses may be suppressed by any particular arachidonic acid metabolite, but a broad range of immune activities are susceptible. The fact that various stimuli may lead to the activation of macrophages, and the subsequent release of suppressive levels of PGE, suggests that this phenomenon may be a rather common event. It is not surprising, therefore, that suppressor macrophages are being described in a variety of immunological systems.

The suppressive activity of PGE, and the suppressive activity of PGE-producing macrophages, are widely accepted today. On the other hand, the indirect activity of PG in modulating Ts cell function is viewed with some skepticism. First, the level of PGE required to induce suppressor cells, described by Webb and his colleagues (54,70-72), ourselves (73) or Fulton and Levy (47), is much higher than would be expected in normal physiological situations. However, current evidence on physiological levels of PGE in an organ such as the spleen do not take into account the microenvironment in which the local concentration of PGE may become significantly elevated. The biological situations which would most likely lead to a possible role for PG induction of suppressor cells would require very high levels of PG and would include various bacterial infections or tumors in which high levels of PG are produced by either macrophages or the tumor cells. Still, questions remain with regard to the biological significance of the PG-induced suppressor cell. For example, what role does the PG-induced suppressor cell play when high levels of immunosuppressive PGE have already been produced?

An additional area of controversy exists with respect to the role of PG synthesis in the mitogen (or antigen)-induced Ts cell. The disagreement which exists in the literature concerning the effect of indomethacin on Con A-induced Ts cells is difficult to reconcile. The studies on SEB-induced Ts cells tend to suggest a role for PG synthesis in the induction phase of these regulatory cells. A question still remains with respect to the relationship between the SEB-Ts cells and antigen-specific Ts cells reported to be induced by various antigens. Additional studies on the role of PG synthesis in the induction of these latter cell populations are warranted. At this time it is clear that Ts cells probably function in complex "circuits" in which more than a single T cell population is required, and several cell-cell interactions take place. Our current studies suggest the possibility that one of these antigen-induced suppressor cell populations may actually be the same population which is activated by SEB. If this is indeed the case, then the role of PG synthesis in the function of these cells would take on much more biological significance.

REFERENCES

1. Webb DR, Nowowiejski I, Healy C, Rogers TJ: Immunosuppressive properties of leukotriene D_4 and E_4 in vitro. Biochem Biophys Res Commun (104): 1617-1622, 1982.
2. Bailey JM, Bryant RW, Low CE, Pupillo MB, Vanderhock JY: Regulation of T-lymphocyte mitogenesis by the leukocyte product 15-hydroxy-eicosatetraenoic acid (15-HETE). Cell Immunol (67): 112-120, 1982.
3. Gualde N, Rabinovitch H, Fredon M, Rigaud M: Effects of 15-hydroperoxyeicosatetraenoic acid on human lymphocyte sheep erythrocyte rosette formation and response to concanavalin A associated with HLA system. Eur J Immunol (12): 773-777, 1982.
4. Payan DG, Goetzl EJ: Specific suppression of human T lymphocyte function by leukotriene B_4. J Immunol (131): 551-553, 1983.
5. Nelson DS: Nonspecific immunoregulation by macrophages and their products. In: Immunobiology of the Macrophage. Academic Press, New York, 1976, pp 235-257.
6. Waldman SR, Gottlier AA: Macrophage regulation of DNA synthesis in lymphoid cells: Effects of a soluble factor from macrophages. Cell Immunol (9): 142-156, 1973.
7. Lopatkin DE, Ranney DF: Maintenance of the resting state and potential regulation of the proliferative phase. In: Lucas DO (ed) Regulatory mechanisms in lymphocyte activation. Academic Press, New York, 1977, pp 195-216.
8. Stobo JD: Immunosuppression in man: Suppression by macrophages can be mediated by interactions with regulatory T cells. J Immunol (119): 918-924, 1977.
9. Pierce CW, Aune TM: Mechanism of action of soluble immune response suppressor. In Hadden J, Mullen P, Chedid L, Sprealico F (ed) Advances in immunopharmacology. Pergammon Press, Oxford, 1981, pp 397-404.
10. Henney CS, Bourne HR, Lichtenstein LM: The role of cyclic 3',5' adenosine monophosphate in the specific cytolytic activity of lymphoyctes. J Immunol (108): 1526-1534, 1972.
11. Strom TB, Carpenter CB, Garovoy MR, Austen KF, Merrill JP, Kaliner M: The modulating influence of cyclic nucleotides upon lymphocyte-mediated cytotoxicity. J Exp Med (138): 381-391, 1973.
12. Darrow TL, Tomar RH: Prostaglandin-mediated regulation of the mixed lymphocyte culture and generation of cytotoxic cells. Cell Immunol (56): 172-183, 1980.

13. Leung KH, Mihich E: Prostaglandin modulation of development of cell-mediated immunity in culture. Nature (288): 597-600, 1980.
14. Hale AH, Evans DL, Daniel LW: Effect of prostaglandins on elicitation of anti-viral cytolytic activity. Immunol Lett (4): 171-174, 1982.
15. Ting C-C, Hargrove ME: Activation of natural killer-derived cytotoxic T lymphocytes. I. Regulation by macrophage and prostaglandins. J Immunol (131): 1734-1741, 1983.
16. Droller MJ, Perlmann P, Schneider MU: Enhancement of natural and antibody-dependent lymphocyte cytotoxicity by drugs which inhibit prostaglandin production by tumor target cells. Cell Immunol (39): 154-164, 1978.
17. Droller MJ, Schneider MU, Perlmann P: A possible role of prostaglandins in the inhibition of natural and antibody-dependent cell-mediated cytotoxicity against tumor cells. Cell Immunol (39): 165-177, 1978.
18. Brunda, MJ, Herberman RB, Holden HT: Inhibition of murine natural killer cell activity by prostaglandins. J Immunol (124): 2682-2687, 1980.
19. Tracey DE, Adkinson NF Jr: Prostaglandin synthesis inhibitors potentiate the BCG-induced augmentation of natural killer cell activity. J Immunol (125) 136-141, 1980.
20. Goto T, Herberman RB, Maluish A, Strong DM: Cyclic AMP as a mediator of prostaglandin E-induced suppression of human natural killer cell activity. J Immunol (130): 1350-1355, 1983.
21. Garovoy MR, Strom TB, Kaliner M, Carpenter CB: Antibody-dependent lymphocyte mediated cytotoxicity mechanism and modulation by cyclic nucleotides. Cell Immunol (20): 197-204, 1975.
22. Wisloff F, Christoffersen T: Role of cyclic nucleotides in human lymphocyte-mediated antibody-dependent cytotoxicity. Int Archs Allergy Appl Immunol (53): 42-49, 1977.
23. Rappaport RS, Dodge GR: Prostaglandin E inhibits the production of human interleukin 2. J Exp Med (155): 943-948, 1982.
24. Tilden AB, Balch CM: A comparison of PGE_2 effects on human suppressor cell function and on interleukin 2 function. J Immunol (129): 2469-2473, 1982.
25. Walker C, Kristensen F, Bettens F, deWeck AL: Lymphokine regulation of activated (G_1) lymphocytes. I. Prostaglandin E_2-induced inhibition of interleukin 2 production. J Immunol (130): 1770-1773, 1983.
26. Gordon D, Bray MA, Morley J: Control of lymphokine secretion by prostaglandins. Nature (262): 401-402, 1976.
27. Koopman WJ, Gillis MH, David JR: Prevention of MIF activity by agents known to increase cellular cyclic AMP. J Immunol (110): 1609-1613, 1973.
28. Metzger Z, Hoffeld JT, Oppenheim JJ: Macrophage-mediated suppression. I. Evidence for participation of both hydrogen peroxide and prostaglandins in suppression of murine lymphocyte proliferation. J Immunol (124): 983-988, 1980.
29. Bourne HR, Lichtenstein LM, Melmon KL, Henney CS, Weinstein Y, Shearer GM: Modulation of inflammation and immunity by cyclic AMP. Science (184): 19-28, 1974.

30. Parker CW, Sullivan TJ, Wedner HJ: Cyclic AMP and the immune response. In Greengard P, Robinson GA (ed) Advances in cyclic nuceotide research. Raven Press, New York, 1974, pp 1-79.
31. DeRubertis FR, Zenser T: Activation of murine lymphocytes by cyclic guanosine 3',5'-monophosphate: Specificity and role in mitogen action. Biochim Biophys Acta (428): 91-103, 1976.
32. DeRubertis FR, Zenser TV, Adler WH, Hudson T: Role of cyclic adenosine 3',5'-monophosphate in lymphocyte mitogenesis. J Immunol (113): 151-161, 1974.
33. Webb DR Jr, Jamieson AT, Nowowiejski I: Control of mitogen-induced transformation: Characterization of a splenic suppressor cell and its mode of action. Cell Immunol (24): 45-57, 1976.
34. Melmon KL, Weinstein Y, Shearer GM, Bourne HR: Leukocyte separation on the basis of their receptors for biogenic amines and prostaglandins: Relation of the receptor to antibody formation. In Braun W, Lichtenstein L, Parker CW (ed) cAMP, cell growth and the immune response. Springer-Verlag New York, New York, 1975, pp 114-134.
35. Plescia OJ, Smith AH, Grinwich K: Subversion of immune systems by tumor cells and role of prostaglandins. Proc Natl Acad Sci USA (72): 1848-1851, 1975.
36. Webb DR, Nowowiejski I: The role of prostaglandins in the control of the primary 19S immune response to sRBC. Cell Immunol (33): 1-10, 1977.
37. Zimecki M, Webb DR: The regulation of the immune response to T-independent antigens by prostaglandins and B cells. J Immunol (117): 2158-2164, 1976.
38. Loose LD, DiLuzio NR: Effect of prostaglandin E_1 on cellular and humoral immune responses. J Reticuloendothel Soc (13): 70-77, 1973.
39. Wieder KJ, Webb DR: The effect of prostaglandin metabolism on immunoglobulin and antibody production in naive and educated whole spleen cells. Prostagland Med (7): 79-90, 1981.
40. Cook RG, Stavitsky AB, Harold WW: Regulation of the in vitro anamnestic antibody response by cyclic AMP. II. Antigen-dependent enhancement by exogenous prostaglandins of the E series. Cell Immunol (40): 128-140, 1978.
41. Gerblich AA, Stavitsky AB: Regulation of the in vitro anamnestic antibody response by cyclic AMP. IV. Evidence for participation of prostaglandins of the E series in the early events. Cell Immunol (48): 318-328, 1979.
42. Kishimoto T, Ishizaka K: Regulation of the antibody response in vitro. X. Biphasic effect of cyclic AMP on the secondary anti-hapten antibody response to anti-immunoglobulin and enhancing soluble factor. J Immunol (116): 534-541, 1976.
43. Gery I, Davies P: Immunoregulatory products of macrophages. In Cohen S, Pick E, Oppenheim J (ed) Biology of the lymphokines. Academic Press, New York, 1979, pp 347-367.
44. Barasoain I, Rojo JM, Portolés A: Effect of indomethacin on in vitro T- and B-cell activation and cell-mediated lysis. Immunopharmacology (2):83-92, 1979.
45. Razin E, Globerson A, Skutelsky E: Indomethacin modulates plasma membrane-associated properties of macrophages. Prostagland Leukotrien Med (8): 301-310, 1982.

46. Atkinson JP, Simchowitz L, Mehta J, Stenson WF: 5,8,11,14-Eicosatetraynoic acid (ETYA) inhibits binding of N-formyl-methionyl-leucyl-phenylalanine (FLMP) to its receptor on human granulocytes. Immunopharmacology (4): 1-9, 1982.
47. Fulton AM, Levy JG: The induction of nonspecific T suppressor lymphocytes by prostaglandin E_1. Cell Immunol (59): 54-60, 1981.
48. Ciosek CP Jr, Ortel RW, Thanassi NM, Newcombe DS: Indomethacin potentiates PGE_1 stimulated cyclic AMP accumulation in human synoviocytes. Nature (251): 148-150, 1974.
49. Newcombe DS, Thanassi NM, Ciosek CP Jr: Cartilage cyclic nucleotide phosphodiesterase: Inhibition by anti-inflammatory agents. Life Sci (14): 505-519, 1974.
50. Jesse RL, Franson RC: Modulation of purified phospholipase A_2 activity from human platelets by calcium and indomethacin. Biochim Biophys Acta (575): 467-470, 1979.
51. Forbes IJ, Smith JL: Effects of anti-inflammatory drugs on lymphocytes. The Lancet (Aug. 12): 334-337, 1967.
52. Siegel MI, McConnell RT, Porter NA, Cuatrecasas, P: Arachidonate metabolism via lipoxygenase and 12L-hydroperoxy-5,8,10,14-icosatetraenoic acid peroxidase sensitive to anti-inflammatory drugs. Proc Natl Acad Sci USA (77): 308-312, 1980.
53. Webb DR, Osheroff PL: Antigen stimulation of prostaglandin synthesis and control of immune responses. Proc Natl Acad Sci USA (73): 1300-1304, 1976.
54. Webb DR, Nowowiejski I: Mitogen-induced changes in lymphocyte prostaglandin levels: A signal for the induction of suppressor cell activity. Cell Immunol (41): 72-85, 1978.
55. Schleimer RP, Benjamini E: Effects of prostaglandin synthesis inhibition on the immune response. Immunopharmacology (3): 205-219, 1981.
56. Barasoain I, Rojo JM, Portolés A: "In vivo" effects of acetylsalicylic acid and two ether derived compounds on primary immune response and lymphoblastic transformation. Immunopharmacology (2): 293-300, 1980.
57. Humes JL, Bonney RJ, Pelus L, Dahlgren ME, Sadowski SJ, Kuehl FA Jr, Davies P: Macrophages synthesise and release prostaglandins in response to inflammatory stimuli. Nature (269): 149-151, 1977.
58. Scott WA, Pawlowski NA, Murray HW, Andreach M, Zrike J, Cohn ZA: Regulation of arachidonic acid metabolism by macrophage activation. J Exp Med (155): 1148-1160, 1982.
59. Bauminger S: Differences in prostaglandin formation between thymocyte subpopulations. Prostaglandins (16): 351-355, 1978.
60. Gemsa D: Stimulation of prostaglandin E release from macrophages and possible role in the immune response. In Pick E (ed) Lymphokines, vol. 4. Academic Press, New York, 1981, pp 335-375.
61. Oropeza-Rendon RL, Ernst M, Schade U, Rietschel ETh, Fischer H: Activation of bone marrow-derived macrophages by repeated zymosan phagocytosis leads to enhanced prostaglandin synthesis. Immunobiology (160): 208-216, 1981.
62. Lapp WS, Mendes M, Kirchner H, Gemsa D: Prostaglandin synthesis by lymphoid tissue of mice experiencing a

graft-versus-host reaction: Relationship to immunosuppression. Cell Immunol (50): 271-281, 1980.
63. Ellner JJ, Spagnuolo PJ: Suppression of antigen and mitogen induced human T lymphocyte DNA synthesis by bacterial lipopolysaccharide: Mediation by monocyte activation and production of prostaglandins. J Immunol (123): 2689-2695, 1979.
64. Mattingly JA, Eardley DD, Kemp JD, Gershon RK: Induction of suppressor cells in rat spleen: Influence of microbial stimulation. J Immunol (122): 787-790, 1979.
65. Mattingly JA, Kemp JD: Suppression of secondary plaque-forming cell responses by rat splenic adherent cells: Evidence for dependence on prostaglandin production. Cell Immunol (48): 195-200, 1979.
66. Kemp J, Louie D, Mattingly J, Bennett J, Higuchi C, Pretell J, Horowitz M, Gershon R: Suppressor cells in vitro: Differential effects of indomethacin and related compounds. J Immunopharmacol (2): 471-489, 1980.
67. Koga Y, Taniguchi K, Kubo C, Nomoto K: Peritoneal adherent cells inhibit the generation of cytotoxic T lymphocytes with prostaglandin-mediated system. Cell Immunol (66): 195-201, 1982.
68. Scott WA, Pawlowski NA, Andreach M, Cohn ZA: Resting macrophages produce distinct metabolites from exogenous arachidonic acid. J Exp Med (155): 535-547, 1982.
69. Folch H, Waksman BH: Regulation of lymphocyte responses in vitro. V. Suppressor activity of adherent and nonadherent rat lymphoid cells. Cell Immunol (9): 12-24, 1973.
70. Rogers TJ, Nowowiejski I, Webb DR: Partial characterization of a prostaglandin-induced suppressor factor. Cell Immunol (50): 82-93, 1980.
71. Webb DR, Wieder K, Rogers TJ, Nowowiejski I: Activation of mouse splenic suppressor cells by endogenous prostaglandin. In de Weck A, Kristensen F, Landy M (ed) Biochemical characterization of lymphokines. Academic Press, New York, 1980, pp 499-501.
72. Webb DR, Rogers TJ, Nowowiejski I: Endogenous prostaglandin synthesis and the control of lymphocyte function. Ann NY Acad Sci (332): 262-270, 1979.
73. Rogers TJ, Campbell L, Calhoun K, Nowowiejski I, Webb DR: Suppression of B-cell and T-cell responses by the prostaglandin-induced T-cell-derived suppressor (PITS). I. Analysis of the $PITS_{\beta}$ factor. Cell Immunol (66): 269-276, 1982.
74. Rogers TJ, O'Day K: A rapid and highly sensitive method of identifying lymphocyte hybridomas by electrophoresis of glucose-phosphate isomerase isozymes. Anal Biochem (116): 389-392, 1981.
75. Rogers TJ, O'Day K: Identification and characterization of lymphocyte hybridomas by electrophoresis of glucose-6-phosphate isomerase isozymes. In Langone JJ, Van Vunakis H (ed) Methods in enzymology, vol. 92. Immunochemical techniques, Part E monoclonal antibodies and general immunoassay methods. Academic Press, New York, 1983, pp 237-242.
76. Jandinski J, Cantor H, Tadakuma T, Peavy DC, Pierce CW: Separation of helper T cells from suppressor T cells express-

ing different Ly components. I. Polyclonal activation: Suppressor and helper activities are inherent properties of distinct T-cell subclasses. J Exp Med (143): 1382-1390, 1976.

77. Tadakuma T, Kühner AL, Rich RR, David JR, Pierce CW: Biological expressions of lymphocyte activation. V. Characterization of a soluble immune response suppressor (SIRS) produced by concanavalin A-activated spleen cells. J Immunol (117): 323-330, 1976.
78. Aune TM, Pierce CW: Mechanism of action of macrophage-derived suppressor factor produced by soluble immune response suppressor-treated macrophages. J Immunol (127): 368-372, 1981.
79. Goodwin JS: Modulation of conconavalin-A-induced suppressor cell activation by prostaglandin E_2. Cell Immunol (49): 421-425, 1980.
80. Skoldstam L, Zoschke D, Messner R: Contrasting effects of prostaglandin E_2 and indomethacin in modulating Con A-induced human lymphocyte proliferation and suppressor cell development. Clin Immunol Immunopathol (25): 32-42, 1982.
81. Soppi E, Eskola J, Ruuskanen O: Effects of indomethacin on lymphocyte proliferation, suppressor cell function, and leukocyte migration inhibitory factor (LMIF) production. Immunopharmacology (4): 235-242, 1982.
82. Badger AM, Griswold DE, Walz DT: Augmentation of concanavalin A-induced immunosuppression by indomethacin. Immunopharmacology (4): 149-162, 1982.
83. Leung KH, Ehrke MJ, Mihich E: Modification by biological products of the generation of suppressor cells in culture. Immunopharmacology (5): 221-237, 1983.
84. Orme IM, Shand FL: Inhibitors of prostaglandin synthetase block the generation of suppressor T cells induced by concanavalin A. Int J Immunopharmacol (3): 15-19, 1981.
85. Orme IM, Shand FL: Concanavalin A-induced alteration of surface marker expression on murine T cells. Int J Immunopharmacol (4): 137-142, 1982.
86. Fischer A, Durandy A, Griscelli C: Role of prostaglandin E_2 in the induction of nonspecific T lymphocyte suppressor activity. J Immunol (126): 1452-1455, 1981.
87. Donnelly RP, Rogers TJ: Immunosuppression induced by Staphylococcal enterotoxin B. Cell Immunol (72): 166-177, 1982.
88. Donnelly RP, Rogers TJ: Inhibitors of prostaglandin synthesis block the induction of Staphylococcal enterotoxin B-activated T-suppressor cells. Cell Immunol (81): 61-70, 1983.
89. Yamamoto I, Webb DR: Antigen-stimulated changes in cyclic nucleotide levels in the mouse. Proc Natl Acad Sci USA (72): 2320-2324, 1975.
90. Winchurch RA, Hilberg C, Birmingham N, Munster AM: Lipopolysaccharide-induced activation of suppressor cells: Reversal by an agent which alters cyclic nucleotide metabolism. Immunology (45): 147-153, 1982.
91. Persson U: Lipopolysaccharide-induced suppression of the primary immune response to a thymus-dependent antigen. J Immunol (118): 789-796, 1977.

92. Koenig S, Hoffman MK: Bacterial lipopolysaccharide activates suppressor B lymphocytes. Proc Natl Acad Sci USA (76): 4608-4612, 1979.
93. Vallera DA, Gamble CE, Schmidtke JR: Lipopolysaccharide-induced immunomodulation of the generation cell-mediated cytotoxicity. II. Evidence for the involvement of a regulatory B lymphocyte. J Immunol (124): 641-649, 1980.

Chapter 5

CONTROL OF ANTIBODY AND AUTOANTIBODY PRODUCTION BY PROSTAGLANDIN E

JAN L. CEUPPENS and JAMES S. GOODWIN

1. INTRODUCTION

In this chapter, we will focus on the effects of prostaglandin E_2 (PGE_2) on humoral immune responses. Results obtained by different authors are often contradictory, making this area confusing but at the same time very exciting. We have studied the influence of PGE_2 on in vitro polyclonal immunoglobulin and rheumatoid factor (RF) production by peripheral blood lymphocytes stimulated with pokeweed mitogen (PWM) and the effects of prostaglandin synthesis inhibition in vivo on serum RF concentrations. Our results indicate that endogenous PGE_2 (produced by monocytes and macrophages) enhances polyclonal immunoglobulin and auto-antibody production through an inhibitory effect on suppressor T cells. In addition to a detailed discussion of our own findings, we will give a survey of the results obtained by other researchers.

2. IN VITRO POLYCLONAL IMMUNOGLOBULIN PRODUCTION

We used an in vitro culture system of human peripheral blood mononuclear cells (PBMC) stimulated with PWM to evaluate the in vitro effect of prostaglandins and prostaglandin synthetase inhibitors on immunoglobulin production (1). Immunoglobulins G and M were measured in the supernatant with an ELISA. PGE_2 was produced in these PWM-stimulated cultures, and the PGE_2 concentration reached a peak after 48 h of about 7 ng/ml. Indomethacin in a dose of 0.5 μg/ml completely suppressed this production (Figure 1). Three different nonsteroidal anti-inflammatory agents (NSAIA) which inhibit cyclooxygenase (indomethacin, carprofen and piroxicam) also suppressed in vitro

J.S. Goodwin (ed.), PROSTAGLANDINS AND IMMUNITY.

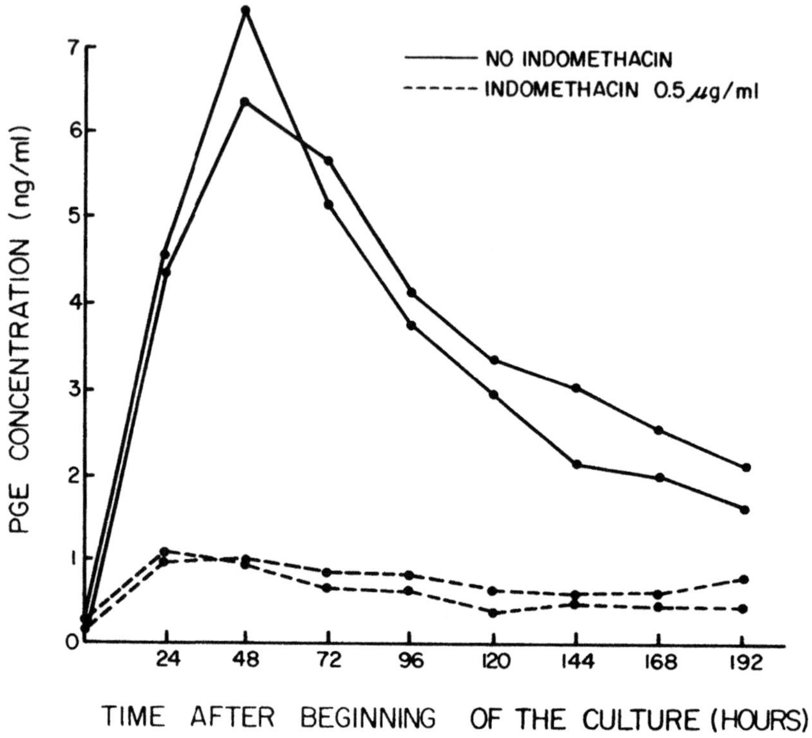

FIGURE 1. PGE_2 production by PBMC (1 x 10^6/ml) stimulated with PWM (1/200) and cultured without or with indomethacin (0.5 µg/ml). Two experiments were performed. Approximately 6-7 ng/ml PGE (2 x 10^{-8}M) was produced after 48 h. [Reproduced from (1) with permission of Cell Immunol.]

immunoglobulin synthesis by about 50% without affecting cell viability. This suggests that an arachidonic acid derivative whose synthesis is blocked by these compounds is required for optimal immunoglobulin production in vitro. The inhibitory effect could be reversed by adding low doses of PGE_2 (3 x 10^{-8} to 3 x 10^{-9}M), which makes PGE_2 the most likely candidate for this function.

There are several possible mechanisms to explain enhancement of polyclonal Ig production by endogenous PGE. The PGE could directly stimulate B cells. It could also stimulate helper T cells, which are required for the B cells to produce Ig. Alternatively, PGE could inhibit suppressor T cells, which tonically suppress the helper T cells. We examined these possibilities in the same in vitro assay system. PGE_2 in concentrations of 3×10^{-9} to 3×10^{-8}M had no effect on purified B cells stimulated with T cell-derived B cell growth and differentiation factors (Table 1). B cells were not directly influenced by PGE_2, except when pharmacological doses were used, which inhibited

Table 1. Effect of PGE_2 on B cells stimulated with helper factor.

	Ig production (ng/ml)	
	IgG	IgM
B cells alone	68 ± 4	<20
B + helper factor	1247 ± 118	947 ± 206
B + helper factor + indomethacin	1201 ± 181	968 ± 114
B + helper factor + indomethacin + PGE^2 3×10^{-9}M	1304 ± 144	892 ± 188
B + helper factor + indomethacin + PGE^2 3×10^{-8}M	1222 ± 93	926 ± 107
B + helper factor + indomethacin + PGE^2 3×10^{-7}M	941 ± 187	740 ± 234
B + helper factor + indomethacin + PGE^2 3×10^{-6}M	318 ± 74	201 ± 45

B cells (E rosette-negative cells depleted of adherent cells on Sephadex G-10) were cultured with 10% helper factor. IgG and IgM production were significantly reduced at both 3×10^{-7}M ($P < 0.05$) and 3×10^{-6}M ($P < 0.001$) by paired t-test. Data are given as means ± SEM for six experiments. Helper factor containing supernatants was prepared by incubating PBMC for 1 h with PWM. Cells were then washed and further incubated for 48 h. After 48 h the supernatants were collected, filtered and stored at -70° C until use. [Reproduced from (1) with permission of Cell Immunol.]

rather than enhanced immunoglobulin production. We therefore hypothesized that the effects of PGE_2 on immunoglobulin production are mediated through regulatory T cells. Irradiation of T cells with 1,000 rads prior to culture completely eliminated the effects of indomethacin and PGE_2. The same loss of effect was observed after mitomycin treatment of the T cells. Both procedures prevented cell proliferation and the generation of suppressor cells. Thus, endogenous PGE_2 produced in the cultures inhibited a radio-sensitive, mitomycin-sensitive suppressor T cell, and suppressor cell control of polyclonal Ig production was itself under negative regulation by endogenous PGE_2. The suppressor cell involved is predominantly but not entirely recognized by OKT8, a monoclonal antibody reacting with T cells of the suppressor-cytotoxic subset (2). Indeed, PGE_2 almost completely inhibits the suppressive activity of OKT8(+) cells added to a culture of B + OKT4(+) helper T cells (Table 2). On the other hand, elimination of OKT8(+) cells reduced but did not entirely eliminate the enhancing effect of PGE_2 on immunoglobulin production. Thomas et al. have shown that some suppressor cells are OKT4(+), which provides a possible explanation for these results (3).

3. INCREASED SENSITIVITY OF SUPPRESSOR T CELLS FROM AGED PEOPLE TO PGE_2

Aging has been associated with increased autoantibody production and decreased suppressor cell function (4,5). T cells of old persons are more sensitive to PGE_2 than T cells from young controls (6). This is also true for suppressor T cells (1). Indomethacin caused significantly greater inhibition of IgG (60 ± 7%) and IgM (58 ± 4%) production in PWM cultures of PBMC from subjects over age 70 than of IgG (44 ± 5%) and IgM (47 ± 3%) production of PBMC from young controls (Figure 2). PGE_2 at different concentrations also induced a significantly greater enhancement of IgG production in lymphocyte cultures from old individuals than from young individuals. These data suggest

Table 2. The target of endogenous PGE_2 is an OKT8(+) T cell.

Cultures	IgM Production (ng/ml)			
	Exp. 1	Exp. 2	Exp. 3	Exp. 4
B + T +				
no drug	4000	...	...	1125
indomethacin	695	...	...	500
indo + PGE	3650	...	...	1675
B + T4(+) +				
no drug	5400	1600	1300	2350
indomethacin	5400	1490	1500	2200
indo + PGE	5780	1540	1450	2625
B + T4(+) + T8(+)				
no drug	2900	975	720	900
indomethacin	1150	510	540	425
indo + PGE	4950	1600	1400	2025

Cultures of B + T cells, B + OKT4(+) T cells and B + OKT4(+) + OKT8(+) cells were established from four subjects. No drug, indomethacin (0.5 µg/ml) or indomethacin plus PGE_2 (3×10^{-8}M) were added. Indomethacin and PGE_2 had little effect on cultures of B + OKT4(+) cells. The addition of PGE to cultures of B + OKT4(+) + OKT8(+) T cells appeared to eliminate the suppression caused by the addition of the OKT8(+) T cells. [Reproduced from (1) with permission of Cell Immunol.]

that one reason for depressed suppressor cell function with age is an increased sensitivity to inhibition by endogenous PGE_2.

4. EFFECT OF PROSTAGLANDINS AND NSAIA ON AUTOANTIBODY PRODUCTION IN VITRO

Human PBMC stimulated with PWM were used to evaluate the in vitro effect of prostaglandins and prostaglandin synthetase inhibitors on IgM-RF production (7). We have previously shown

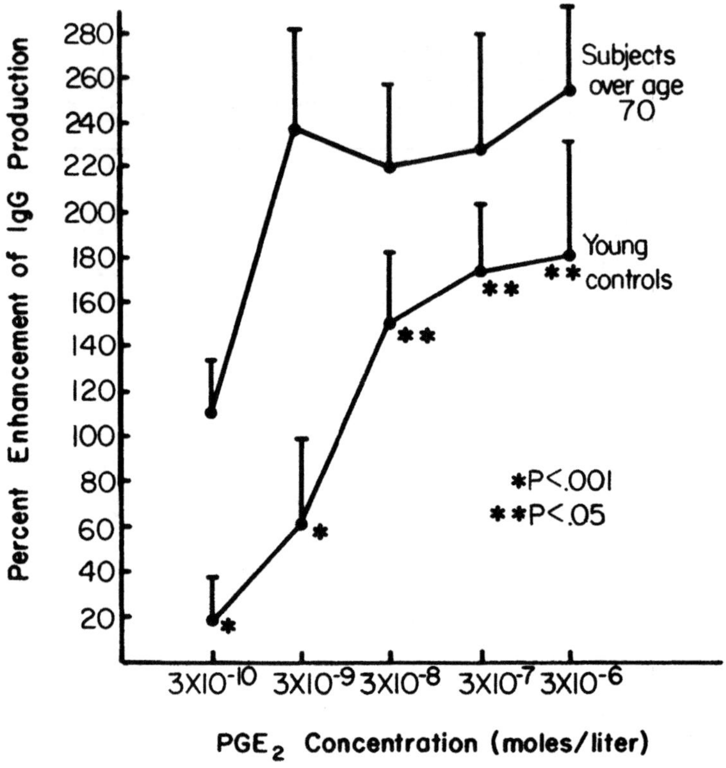

FIGURE 2. Enhancement of IgG production by PGE_2 in PWM-stimulated cultures of lymphocytes from subjects over 70 and young controls. Different concentrations of PGE_2 were added to cultures containing indomethacin. Results are expressed as the mean (± SEM) percentage enhancement for 12 subjects over 70 and 12 young controls run in parallel with the old subjects. There was significantly greater enhancement by each concentration of PGE_2 of IgG production by lymphocytes from subjects over 70. Data were analysed by paired t-test. [Reproduced from (1) with permission of Cell Immunol (1).]

that in this system, OKT4(+) helper T cells are needed for RF production, while OKT8(+) cells suppress the RF production (8). Figure 3 summarizes some in vitro studies in which we measured the effect of NSAIA on the production of IgM-RF by lymphocytes from patients with rheumatoid arthritis. One million lymphocytes from these patients were cultured with PWM for 1 wk, and

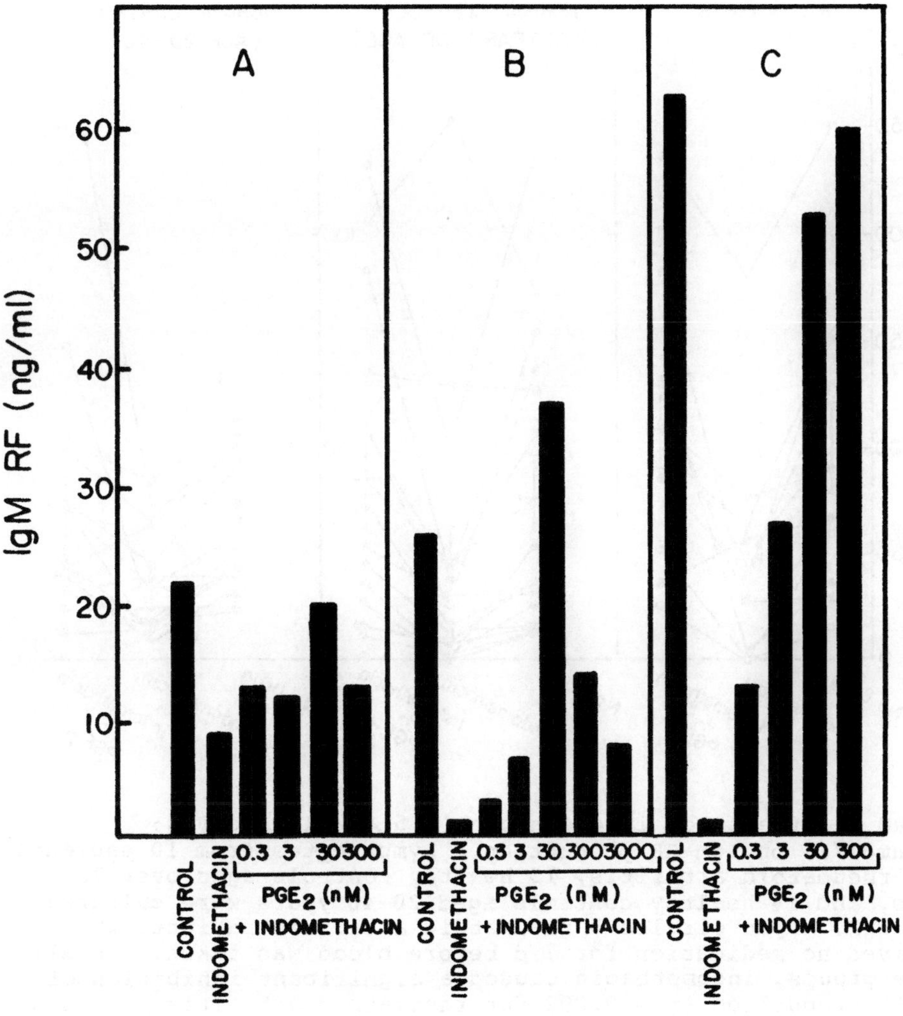

FIGURE 3. Effect of addition of different concentrations of PGE_2 on IgM-RF production. In three experiments with PWM-stimulated lymphocyte cultures, indomethacin (0.5 µg/ml) caused substantial inhibition of IGM-RF production. This was reversed by adding PGE_2 (0.3 to 3,000 nmol/l) to the cultures. [Reproduced from (7) with permission of Lancet.]

the production of IgM-RF in the supernate was measured with a radioimmunoassay. When indomethacin was added to the culture, the RF production was inhibited, and then as PGE_2 was readded

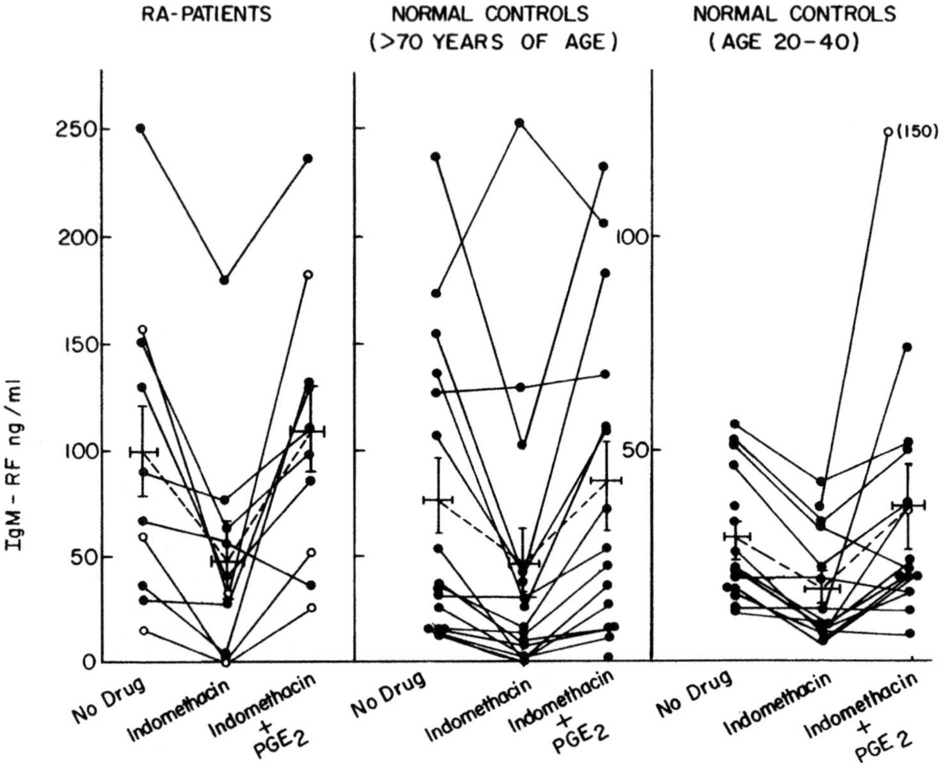

FIGURE 4. Effects of indomethacin (0.5 μg/ml) and PGE_2 (30 nmol/l) on IgM-RF production. Lymphocytes from 10 patients with rheumatoid arthritis, 15 healthy controls aged over 70 years, and 14 healthy controls aged 20-40 years were cultured with PWM. Open circles = rheumatoid arthritis patients who received no medication for 7 d before blood was taken. In all three groups, indomethacin caused a significant inhibition of IgM-RF production ($p = 0.002$ for rheumatoid arthritis patients, $p = 0.02$ for controls over 70 years, and $p = 0.0001$ for controls aged 20-40 years, by paired t-test). Addition of 30 nmol/l PGE_2 caused a significant enhancement in IgM-RF production over the level with indomethacin ($p = 0.003$ for rheumatoid arthritis patients, $p = 0.01$ for controls over 70 years, and $p = 0.02$ for controls aged 20-40 years). [Reproduced from (7) with permission of Lancet.]

to these cultures with indomethacin, IgM-RF gradually increased to control levels. In all three cases, it can be seen that the amount of PGE_2 required to restore the RF levels to control values was approximately 30 nM. Figure 4 provides a summary of experiments on patients with rheumatoid arthritis and also on young and old healthy donors whose lymphocytes produce RF. It can be seen that the addition of indomethacin lowers the production of RF, and the readdition of PGE_2 at 3 to 30 nM restores RF production to the control values. As can be seen in Table 3, three different NSAIA tested in vitro in concentrations found in the sera of patients taking these agents all inhibited RF production. This gives further evidence for the fact that the effect observed was due to inhibition of arachidonic acid metabolism. The mechanism of this inhibition was further examined. Irradiating T cells prior to culture eliminated the inhibitory effect of NSAIA and the stimulatory effect of PGE_2 (Table 4). This suggests that endogenous prostaglandin was inhibiting a radiosensitive suppressor T cell. We tested this more directly by separating helper and supppressor T cells with monoclonal antibodies. Once again, when B + T cells were cultured, indomethacin inhibited and prostaglandin stimulated RF production. However, when B cells were cultured with isolated OKT4(+) helper T cells, indomethacin no longer inhibited and PGE_2 no longer stimulated. When suppressor cells, identified by the OKT8 monoclonocal antibody, were added back to this system, then once again indomethacin inhibited and PGE_2

Table 3. Effect of nonsteroidal anti-inflammatory agents on IgM-RF production in vitro by lymphocytes from patients with rheumatoid arthritis.

Drug	Percent Inhibition
Indomethacin (0.5 µg/ml)	55%
Indomethacin (5.0 µg/ml)	44%
Carprofen (10 µg/ml)	60%
Piroxicam (10 µg/ml)	80%

Results are expressed as percent inhibition of IgM-RF production in comparison to cultures with no drugs. Drug concentrations used were comparable to serum concentrations in patients taking the drugs. [Adapted from (7).]

Table 4. Inhibition by indomethacin and stimulation by PGE_2 of IgM-RF production requires the presence of a radiosensitive T cell.

	IgM-RF production (ng/ml)		
	No drugs	Indomethacin (0.5 μg/ml)	Indomethacin + PGE_2 (30 nM/l)
B + T	48 ± 22	13 ± 5	47 ± 21
B + T (1,000 rad)	45 ± 17	37 ± 16	34 ± 8

Results are the means ± SEM of six experiments. In B + T cultures, indomethacin caused a 73% inhibition of IgM-RF production, which was completely reversed by PGE_2 (comparing cultures with no drugs with cultures plus indomethacin, $p < 0.01$; comparing cultures plus indomethacin with cultures plus indomethacin and PGE_2, $p < 0.01$ by paired t-test). In the B(+) irradiated T cultures, indomethacin caused a slight (18%), but not significant, inhibition of IgM-RF production, and addition of PGE_2 had no effect. [Reproduced from (7) with permission of Lancet.]

stimulated RF production. Thus, PGE_2 inhibits a radiosensitive OKT8(+) suppressor cell, whose function is to suppress autoantibody formation.

5. EFFECT OF NSAIA ON AUTOANTIBODY PRODUCTION IN VIVO

To test the validity of our hypothesis for the in vivo situation, we placed 20 patients with rheumatoid arthritis on a cyclooxygenase inhibitor (piroxicam) (9). All 20 patients had been on one or another NSAIA prior to the study. They were then placed on placebo medication and the NSAIA were stopped for 2 wk. In all cases, serum RF levels rose. The patients were then placed on piroxicam 20 mg once a day for 10 wk. The RF levels quickly went back to control and continued to decrease throughout the 10 wk length of the study ($P < 0.001$ by paired t-test for each comparison) (Figure 5). In addition, the percentage of OKT8(+) suppressor cells within the E-Rosette (+) lymphocyte population was found to increase during treatment. We conclude from these data that our in vitro findings are also

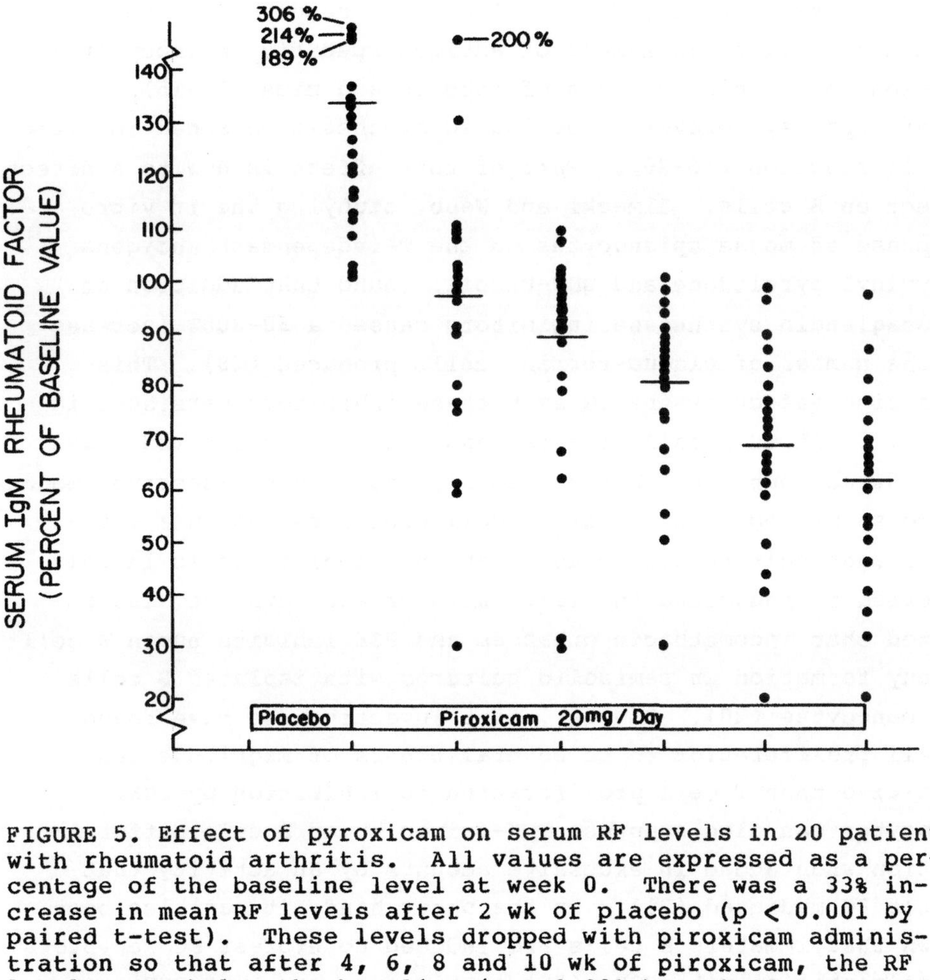

FIGURE 5. Effect of pyroxicam on serum RF levels in 20 patients with rheumatoid arthritis. All values are expressed as a percentage of the baseline level at week 0. There was a 33% increase in mean RF levels after 2 wk of placebo ($p < 0.001$ by paired t-test). These levels dropped with piroxicam administration so that after 4, 6, 8 and 10 wk of piroxicam, the RF levels were below the baseline ($p < 0.001$ by paired t-test for each comparison). [Reproduced from (9) with permission of JAMA.]

relevant for the in vivo situation, and that PGE_2 represents a negative feedback mechanism for suppressor cell control of autoantibody formation.

6. OTHER STUDIES ON THE EFFECTS OF PGE_2 ON ANTIBODY PRODUCTION IN VITRO

Several groups have reported similar findings to ours that PGE_2 stimulates and/or cyclooxygenase inhibitors depress the production of immunoglobulin in polyclonally stimulated cultures of human lymphocytes (10-12). Analogous results have been obtained in vitro in assays of antigen-specific antibody production in splenic cultures of rabbits and mice (13-15). In other reports, however, blocking PG synthesis enhanced in vitro B cell function (16-20). Part of this effect is due to a direct effect on B cells. Zimecki and Webb, studying the in vitro response of mouse splenocytes to the T-independent antigens polyvinyl pyrolidone and DNP-Ficoll, found that addition of prostaglandin synthetase inhibitors caused a 50-300% increase in the number of plaque-forming cells produced (18). This enhancing effect of the PG synthetase inhibitors persisted in highly purified B cell preparations with no T cells and fewer than 5% macrophages. Kurland et al. found that excessive amounts of mouse macrophages inhibit B cell proliferation in a semisolid agar culture system and that this inhibition is largely reversed by indomethacin (19). Whisler and Newhouse also reported that indomethacin enhances and PGE inhibits human B cell colony formation in semisolid cultures with isolated B cells and monocytes (20). However, most investigators have found B cell proliferation to be several orders of magnitude less sensitive than T cell proliferation to inhibition by PGE. Monocytes can also suppress PWM-driven human B cell differentiation when added in excessive amounts by an activity that is not PG mediated (21). On the other hand, it has also been shown that immature B cells are induced to express Fc receptors upon incubation with PGE_2 (22). This suggests that PGE_2 can induce differentiation of immature B cells, while it inhibits further proliferation and plasma cell differentiation. In another study, the effect of indomethacin in vitro was found to be due to enhanced helper T cell function: Webb and Nowowiejski reported that the helper activity of thymocytes incubated with sheep red blood cells (RBC) for 24 h was enhanced when indomethacin was also present during this preincubation phase (16). On the other hand, Emilie et al. reported that preincubation of T cells with PGE_2 enhanced the helper activity for an antigen-specific antibody response against TNP-polyacrylamide beads.

This stimulatory effect of PGE_2 on helper cells could be neutralized by a nondialysable monocyte factor (23). Delfraissy et al. (24) reported that the abolished in vitro antibody response of PBMC from subjects over age 70 to TNP could be completely restored to normal (young) levels by addition of indomethacin or removal of glass-adherent cells. These investigators also found that lymphocytes from aged people were much more sensitive to PGE_2 than lymphocytes from young controls. The target of PGE activity was not clearly identified in these studies.

Several authors have studied the effect of PGE on suppressor cell function in relation to Ig production. Our results suggested that endogenous PGE tonically suppresses a radiosensitive, OKT8(+) suppressor T cell of polyclonal immunoglobulin and RF production in PWM-stimulated cultures of human lymphocytes. Other laboratories have reported that PGE inhibits and indomethacin stimulates concanavalin A (Con A)-activated suppressor cell generation in vitro (25-28), which agrees with our data. The concept that NSAIA, by blocking PGE production, may enhance suppressor T cell function in patients with rheumatoid arthritis has received additional support from the recent work of Hasler and associates (29). T lymphocytes from patients with rheumatoid arthritis have an impaired ability to suppress B lymphocyte activation by Epstein Barr Virus (EBV) (30). This inability to generate suppressor cells in vitro can be corrected by the addition of indomethacin to the cultures (29). It would appear that a subset of lymphocytes from patients with rheumatoid arthritis is exquisitely sensitive to endogenous PGE and that this increased sensitivity to PGE is responsible for the defect in EBV-specific suppressor cell induction. Tγ cells have been shown by Moretta et al. to be suppressive for PWM-driven B cell differentiation into plasma cells (31). T cells bearing a receptor for the Fc portion of IgG (Tγ cells) had a 27-fold rise in cyclic AMP after exposure to PGE_2, whereas the remaining T cells had a four-fold increase (32). Thus, Tγ cells have a high density of PGE_2 receptors on their membranes relative to non-Tγ cells. This rise in cyclic AMP can either be an inhibition or an activation signal, and functional studies are needed to differentiate between these possibilities.

There is, indeed, also considerable evidence that PGE participates in activation of T suppressor cells. For example, Webb and coworkers showed that PGE_2 activates a glass-adherent suppressor T cell in mouse spleen to release two peptides which in turn suppress the response of nonadherent T cells to mitogens (33-35). This suppressor factor also inhibits the antibody response to both T-dependent and T-independent antigens (35). The authors conclude that the inhibition by PGE of immune responses is directly mediated via activation of suppressor cells. However, the concentration of PGE_2 needed to induce the suppressor factor was very high: 10^{-5}M. Fisher et al. demonstrated that small concentrations of PGE_2 (10^{-9}M) are a necessary but not sufficient component of the generation of human Con A-activated suppressor cells (36). Addition of indomethacin or anti-PGE antibodies to the Con A-stimulated cultures blocked generation of suppressor cells, and the generation of suppressor cells could be restored by adding back 10^{-9}M PGE to the cultures. Addition of PGE at 10^{-9}M alone, without Con A, did not result in generation of suppressor cells. However, higher concentrations of PGE_2 (10^{-7}M) were able to induce suppressor T cells by themselves. Durandy et al. investigated B cell differentiation in non-immunodeficient children receiving gammaglobulin injections and found a defect in B cell differentiation secondary to increased suppressor T cell activity (37). These suppressor cells could also be induced in vitro by exposure of normal lymphocytes to gammaglobulin preparations. This in vitro generation of suppressor T cells was dependent on PGE_2 production.

It would appear that in addition to being directly inhibitory of suppressor T cell function, PGE is required in the generation and/or action of other types of suppressor T cells. Further studies are needed to evaluate the relative importance and specificity of these opposing effects.

7. EFFECT OF NSAIA ON ANTIGEN-SPECIFIC ANTIBODY PRODUCTION IN VIVO

Webb and Osheroff were the first to demonstrate that inhibition of immune function by endogenous prostaglandins represents a physiologic feedback mechanism (38). These authors found that injection of mice with sheep RBC led to an 80-fold increase in intrasplenic prostaglandin $F_2\gamma$. Prior administration of a PG synthetase inhibitor prevented the PG increase and also resulted in a significantly increased number of plaque-forming spleen cells 3 to 5 d after sensitization. Thus, prostaglandin synthetase inhibitors seem to enhance humoral immune responses in vivo. Goodwin et al. examined the effect of indomethacin administration on humoral immunity in man by administering indomethacin (100 mg/d) to 15 normal subjects from 2 d before until 10 d after they received a bivalent influenza vaccine (39). Compared to 15 age and sex matched controls, the indomethacin-treated group had a significantly increased antibody titer to A-Victoria ($P < 0.02$). There was no difference in titer to A-New Jersey. Since 90% of the subjects had antibody titers to A-Victoria prior to vaccination, while none had prior titers to A-New Jersey, the results suggested that indomethacin administration enhanced the secondary but not the primary humoral immune response. Garin and Richard reported that indomethacin normalized the antibody response to sheep RBC in rats with experimental nephrotic syndrome. These rats also had increased plasma levels of 6-keto $PGF_2\alpha$ before treatment. Indomethacin had no effect on the antibody response in normal rats (40).

The effects of NSAIA on antigen-specific antibody production in vivo thus are quite different from the effects on autoantibody production in vivo, as reported in our study on RF production. This suggests different suppressor cell control mechanisms for antigen-specific antibody production and autoantibody production. Kelley and associates have studied the effects of PGE administration on strains of mice that spontaneously develop lupus-like glomerulonephritis. PGE was found to suppress the immune response and antibody production to retroviral gp70, resulting in decreased amounts of gp70-anti-gp70 immune complexes, retarded glomerular deposition of immune complexes and prolonged survival. PGE had little effect on anti-DNA antibodies (41). Thus, these authors found an inhibition of antigen-specific antiviral antibodies, while auto-antibodies were unchanged. NSAIA, on the other hand, did not influence anti-DNA or anti-gp70 antibodies (42).

As to the mechanism of enhanced antibody production after administration of cyclooxygenase inhibitors in vivo, it has been suggested that these compounds inhibit suppressor cell generation in vivo. Shimamura and coworkers have shown that indomethacin administration to mice blocks generation of antigen-specific splenic suppressor cells in vivo following immunization with a high dose of sheep RBC (43). Badger et al. also reported that in vivo administration of indomethacin to mice blocks suppressor T cell generation by Con A of the in vitro antibody response to sheep RBC (28).

8. DISCUSSION

By far the most confusing area of research on PGE and immunity is comprised of those experiments dealing with the regulation of immunoglobulin production and suppressor cell function by PGE. Not only have seemingly conflicting results been reported by different groups using different assay systems, but directly contradictory results have been reported by different groups using the same assay system. In some instances, both sets of contradictory data have been reproduced by yet other groups. There is an understandable temptation for anyone confronting such disarray to dismiss all the experimental findings in this area as meaningless, or at least as uninterpretable. We feel that this would be a mistake; there is "truth" lurking out there that will become apparent when all investigators in the field pay scrupulous attention to the minor methodologic details (such as the choice of round bottom vs. flat bottom microwells, or such as letting the cells sit overnight during a long experimental protocol) that may have major effects on regulation by PGE. The student of this literature must be a critical reader, paying particular attention to dosages of the agents used. To give just two examples, doses of indomethacin that are safe in humans (1-3 mg/kg/d) will cause a wasting disease in many types of rodents. Also, mouse splenocytes in culture are often very sensitive to the traces of ethanol sometimes used to solubilize the drugs, while human lymphocytes are unaffected by much higher levels. In addition to these potentially confounding methodological problems, there are many other difficulties which arise from the grossness of the tools we use to examine prostaglandins. We cannot inhibit PGE production in only one tissue in the body or in only one cell type in a culture; indeed, we cannot even specifically inhibit PGE production without also inhibiting the other cyclooxygenase metabolites as well as the 15-lipoxygenase products. Using in vitro models, it is possible to block all cyclooxygenase products by, for example, indomethacin, and then to show that the effect observed is mediated by a particular metabolite, such as PGE_2, by adding back this metabolite to the culture system. We have used this method in our in vitro studies (1,7). However, the problem is more complicated for in vivo studies with NSAIA, since it is impossible to substitute for particular metabolites.

Based on our in vitro studies, we propose the following model for regulation of polyclonal immunoglobulin and autoantibody production by prostaglandins (Figure 6). The B cells produce RF with the help of T helper cells. In this system, T suppressor cells would normally shut off the T helper cells, resulting in no autoantibody production (8). However, PGE_2 produced by the monocytes tonically inhibits suppressor cell activity. Thus, the suppressor cells are shut off, allowing the T helper cells to help the B cells make RF. When a NSAIA is added to the system, it shuts off PGE production, allowing the suppressor cells to grow up and shut off helper cell function, resulting in decreased RF production. While endogenous PGE_2 stimulates RF production in vitro, it is not certain that

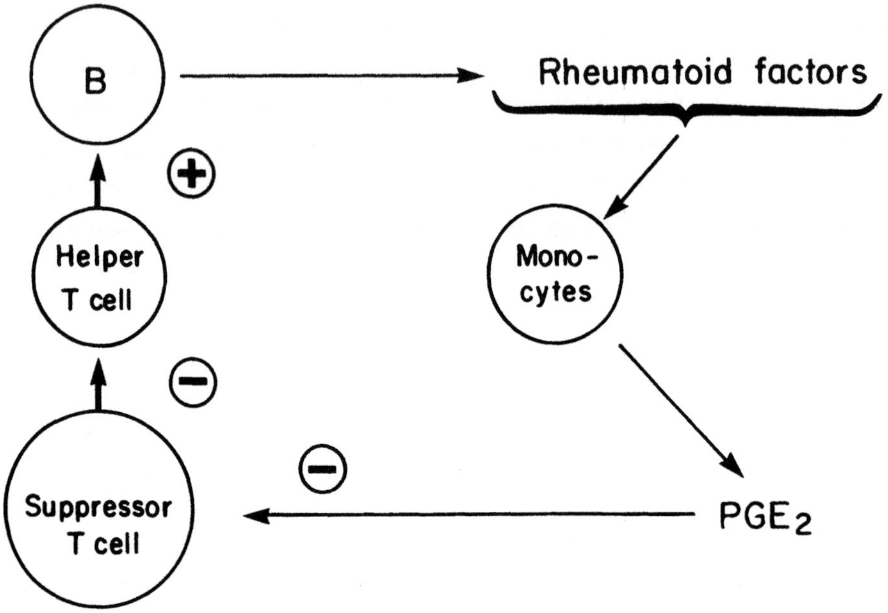

FIGURE 6. Outline of mechanisms whereby NSAIA inhibit RF production.

PGs have a comparable role in vivo. The levels of PGs that are produced in the test tube (approximately 10^{-8}M) are 100 to 1,000 times higher than are found in the sera of patients with rheumatoid arthritis or normal controls. However, it is interesting to note that high concentrations of prostaglandin are found in the synovial fluid of rheumatoid joints (44). These high local concentrations of prostaglandin may explain why RF is preferentially produced in the rheumatoid joint. Thus, the prostaglandin can selectively shut off suppressor cell function in the joint, resulting in local RF production. However, in peripheral tissues with normal concentrations of prostaglandin, suppressor cell function remains normal. This model is supported by our observation that NSAIA administration in vivo decreased RF serum levels and increased the number of OKT8 cells (9). In addition, in two very different in vitro assay systems, RF production and EBV-stimulated B cell proliferation, NSAIA have been shown to stimulate suppressor cell function and thereby partially to correct basic immunoregulatory disturbances in the disease (7,29).

Many diseases, as discussed in other chapters, are characterized by an increased production of PGE_2 by "prostaglandin producing suppressor cells," e.g., coccidiomycosis (45), rheumatoid arthritis (46,47), experimental cutaneous leishmaniasis (48), tuberculosis(49), Chagas' disease (50), filariasis (51), sarcoidosis (52) and Hodgkin's disease (53). In many of these diseases, depressed cellular immune function is accompanied by polyclonal hypergammaglobulinemia. Both effects can be explained by increased PGE_2 production, which is itself secondary to chronic immune stimulation. PGE_2, on the one hand, induces decreased mitogen responsiveness and T cell function, while inhibition of non-specific suppressor T cells leads to hypergammaglobulinemia. Antigen-specific antibody production, however, does not seem to be under the same control mechanism. Both human and animal studies suggest an enhancement of antigen-specific antibody production by NSAIA. This cannot be explained by an inhibitory effect of PGE_2 on suppressor cells. Therefore, further studies are needed to confirm these findings, while animal models or a system with in vitro antigen-specific suppressor cell generation and antibody production are needed to elucidate the mechanism.

REFERENCES

1. Ceuppens J, Goodwin JS: Endogenous prostaglandin E enhances polyclonal immunoglobulin production by tonically inhibiting T suppressor cell activity. Cell Immunol (70): 41-54, 1982.
2. Reinherz EL, Schlossman SF: Regulation of the immune response: inducer and suppressor T-lymphocyte subsets in human beings. N Engl J Med (303): 370-373, 1980.
3. Thomas Y, Rogozinski L, Irigoyen O, Friedman SM, Kung PC, Goldstein G, Chess L: Functional analysis of human T cell subsets defined by monoclonal antibodies. IV. Induction of suppressor cells within the OKT_4(+) population. J Exp Med (154): 459-467, 1981.

4. Hallgren HM, Yunis EJ: Suppressor lymphocytes in young and aged humans. J Immunol (118): 1004-1009, 1977.
5. Kishimoto S, Tomino S, Mitsuya H, Fujiwara H: Age-related changes in suppressor cell functions of human T-cells. J Immunol (123): 1586-1591, 1979.
6. Goodwin JS, Messner RP: Sensitivity of lymphocytes to prostaglandin E_2 increases in subjects over 70 years of age. J Clin Invest (64): 434-439, 1979.
7. Ceuppens JL, Goodwin JS: Non-steroidal anti-inflammatory agents inhibit the synthesis of IgM rheumatoid factor in vitro. Lancet (1): 528-533, 1982.
8. Rodriguez MA, Ceuppens JL, Goodwin JS: Regulation of IgM rheumatoid factor production in lymphocyte cultures from young and old subjects. J Immunol (128): 2422-2428, 1982.
9. Goodwin JS, Ceuppens JL, Rodriguez MA: Effect of nonsteroidal anti-inflammatory agents on immunologic function in patients with rheumatoid arthritis. JAMA (250): 2485-2488, 1983.
10. Panayi GS, Staite ND, Unger A: Indomethacin inhibits in vitro immunoglobulin production by human B lymphocytes. Agents Actions (11): 608-610, 1981.
11. Lydyard PM, Brostoff J, Hudspith B, Parry H: Prostaglandin E_2-mediated enhancement of human plasma cell differentiation. Immunol Lett (4): 113-116, 1982.
12. Staite ND, Panayi GS: Regulation of human immunoglobulin production in vitro by prostaglandin E_2. Clin Exp Immunol (49): 115-122, 1982.
13. Gerblich AA, Stavitsky AB: Regulation of the in vitro anamnestic antibody response by cAMP. IV. Evidence for participation of prostaglandins of the E series in the early events. Cell Immunol (48): 318-328, 1979.
14. Cook R: Regulation of the in vitro anamnestic antibody response by cyclic AMP. II. Prostaglandins of the E series. Cell Immunol (40): 128-133, 1978.
15. Wieder KJ, Webb DR: The effect of prostaglandin metabolism on immunoglobulin and antibody production in naive and educated whole spleen cells. Prost Med (7): 79-90, 1981.
16. Webb DR, Nowowiejski I: The role of prostaglandins in the control of the primary immune response to sRBC. Cell Immunol (33): 1-10, 1977.
17. Mattingly JA, Kemp JD: Suppression of secondary plaque-forming cell responses by rat splenic adnerent cells; evidence for dependence on prostaglandin production. Cell Immunol (48): 195-201, 1979.
18. Zimecki M, Webb DR: The regulation of the immune response to T-independent antigens by prostaglandins and B cells. J Immunol (117): 2158-2164, 1976.
19. Kurland JI, Kincade PW, Moore MAS: Regulation of B lymphocyte clonal proliferation by stimulatory and inhibitory macrophage-derived factors. J Exp Med (146): 1420-1427, 1977.
20. Wisler RL, Newhouse YG: Inhibition of human B lymphocyte colony responses by endogenous synthetised hydrogen peroxide and prostaglandins. Cell Immunol (69): 34-45, 1982.

21. Gmelig-Myerling F, Waldmann T: Human B cell activation in vitro: augmentation and suppression by monocytes of the immunoglobulin production induced by various B-cell stimulants. J Immunol (126): 529-536, 1981.
22. Burchiel SW, Warner NL: Cyclic AMP modulation of Fc receptor expression on a pre-B cell lymphoma. J Immunol (124):1016-1021, 1980.
23. Emilie D, Crevon MC, Galanaud P: Prostaglandin E_2 regulation of human specific B-cell response: interaction with a monocyte product. Clin Immunol Immunopathol (29): 415-423, 1983.
24. Delfraissy JF, Garanaud P, Wallon C, Balavoine JF, Dormont J: Abolished in vitro antibody response in elderly: exclusive involvement of prostaglandin-induced T suppressor cells. Clin Immunol Immunopathol (24): 377-385, 1982.
25. Goodwin JS: Modulation of concanavalin A-induced suppressor cell activation by prostaglandin E_2. Cell Immunol (49): 421-425, 1980.
26. Skoldstam L, Zoschke D, Messner R: Increase in Con A-induced suppressor cell activity after indomethacin treatment. Arthritis Rheum (25): 357-359, 1982.
27. Skoldstam L, Zoschke D, Messner R: Contrasting effects of prostaglandin E_2 and indomethacin in modulating Con A-induced human lymphocyte proliferation and suppressor cell development. Clin Immunol Immunopathol (25): 32-42, 1982.
28. Badger AM, Griswold DE, Walz DT: Augmentation of concanavalin A-induced immunosuppression by indomethacin. Immunopharmacol (4): 149-162, 1982.
29. Hasler F, Bluestein HG, Zvaifler NJ, Epstein LB: Analysis of the defects responsible for the impaired regulation of EBV-induced B cell proliferation by rheumatoid arthritis lymphocytes. II. Role of monocytes and the increased sensitivity of rheumatoid arthritis lymphocytes to prostaglandin E. J Immunol (131): 768-772, 1983.
30. Tosato G, Steinberg AD, Blaese RM: Defective EB virus-specific suppressor cell function in rheumatoid arthritis. N Engl J Med (305): 1238-1244, 1981.
31. Moretta L, Webb DR, Grossi CE, Lydyard PM, Cooper MD: Functional analysis of two human T-cell subpopulations: help and suppression of B-cell responses by T-cell bearing receptors for IgM or IgG. J Exp Med (146): 194-199, 1977.
32. Goodwin JS, Kaszubowski PA, Williams RC Jr: Cyclic adenosine monophosphate response to prostaglandin E_2 in subpopulations of human lymphocytes. J Exp Med (150): 1260-1267, 1979.
33. Webb DR, Nowowiejski I: Mitogen-induced changes in lymphocyte prostaglandin levels: a signal for the induction of suppressor cell activity. Cell Immunol (41): 72-78, 1978.
34. Rogers TJ, Nowowiejski I, Webb DR: Partial characterization of a prostaglandin-induced suppressor factor. Cell Immunol (50): 82-89, 1980.
35. Rogers TJ, Campbell L, Calhoon K, Nowowiejski I, Webb DR: Suppression of B-cell and T-cell responses by the prostaglandin induced T cell derived suppressor (PITS). Cell Immunol (66): 269-276, 1982.

36. Fisher A, Durandy A, Griscelli C: Role of prostaglandin E_2 in the induction of nonspecific T lymphocyte suppressor activity. J Immunol (126): 1452-1455, 1981.
37. Durandy A, Fisher A, Griscelli C: Dysfunctions of pokeweed mitogen-stimulated T and B lymphocyte responses induced by gammaglobulin therapy. J Clin Invest (67): 867-877, 1981.
38. Webb DR, Osheroff PL: Antigen stimulation of prostaglandin synthesis and control of immune response. Proc Natl Acad Sci USA (73): 1300-1309, 1976.
39. Goodwin JS, Selinger DS, Messner RP, Reed WP: Effect of indomethacin in vivo on humoral and cellular immunity in humans. Infect Immun (19): 430-437, 1978.
40. Garin EH, Richard GA: Prostaglandin synthesis inhibition and primary antibody response in experimental nephrotic syndrome. Clin Immunol Immunopathol (30): 129-133, 1984.
41. Izui S, Kelley V, McConahey PJ, Dixon FJ: Selective suppression of retroviral gp70-anti-gp70 immune complex formation by prostaglandin E_1 in immune systemic lupus erythematosus. J Exp Med (152): 1645-1658, 1980.
42. Kelley VE, Izui S, Halushka PV: Effect of Ibuprofen, a fatty acid cyclooxygenase inhibitor, on murine lupus. Clin Immunol Immunopathol (25): 223-231, 1982.
43. Shimamura T, Hashimoto K, Sasaki S: Feedback suppression of the immune response in vivo. II. Involvement of prostaglandins in the generation of suppressor-inducer B lymphocytes. Cell Immunol (69): 192-195, 1982.
44. Robinson DR, Levine L: Prostaglandin concentrations in synovial fluid in rheumatic diseases: action of indomethacin and aspirine. In: Robinson HJ, Vane JR (eds): Prostaglandin synthetase inhibitors. Raven Press, New York, 1975, pp 223-228.
45. Catanzaro A: Suppressor cells in coccidiomycosis. Cell Immunol (64): 235-245, 1981.
46. Wolinsky S, Goodwin JS, Messner RP, Williams RC Jr: Role of prostaglandin in the depressed cell-mediated immune response in rheumatoid arthritis. Clin Immunol Immunopathol (17): 31-36, 1980.
47. Seitz M, Deimann W, Gram N, Huntstein W, Gemsa D: Characterization of blood mononuclear cells of rheumatoid arthritis patients. Clin Immunol Immunopathol (25): 405-416, 1982.
48. Scott PA, Farrell JP: Experimental cutaneous leishmaniasis. J Immunol (127): 2395-2400, 1981.
49. Kleinhenz ME, Ellner J, Spagnuolo PJ, Daniel TM: Suppression of lymphocyte responses by tuberculous plasma and mycobacterial arabinogalactan. J Clin Invest (68): 153-162, 1981.
50. Kierszenbaum F: Immunologic deficiency during experimental Chagas' disease (trypanosoma cruzi infection). J Immunol (129): 2202-2205, 1982.
51. Piessens WF, Partono F, Hoffman SL, Ratiwayanto S, Piessens PW, Palmieri JR, Koiman I, Dennis DT, Carney WP: Antigen-specific suppressor T lymphocytes in human lymphatic filariasis. N Engl J Med (307): 144-148, 1982.

52. Goodwin JS, DeHoratius R, Israel H, Peake GT, Messner RP: Suppressor cell function in sarcoidosis. Ann Intern Med (90): 169-175, 1979.
53. Goodwin JS, Messner RP, Bankhurst AD, Peake GT, Saiki JH, Wiliams RC Jr: Prostaglandin-producing suppressor cells in Hodgkin's disease. N Engl J Med (197): 263-269, 1977.

Chapter 6

EFFECTS OF PROSTAGLANDINS ON IN VIVO IMMUNE AND INFLAMMATORY REACTIONS

Joseph C. Fantone, Steven L. Kunkel and Robert B. Zurier

INTRODUCTION

The initial observation of Kloeze in the 1960's (1) that a metabolite of arachidonic acid, prostaglandin E (PGE), inhibited platelet aggregation led to the notion that cyclooxygenase products of arachidonic acid metabolism might have antiinflammatory activity. Subsequent studies demonstrating the ability of prostacyclin (PGI_2) and PGE_1 to inhibit platelet aggregation both in vitro and in vivo, and the production of relatively large quantities of PGI_2 by endothelial cells served as a basis for defining one of the most important regulatory mechanisms involved in the initiation and progression of thrombus formation (reviewed in 2). Consequences of thrombosis (i.e. ischemia and infarction) are well known and serve as a basis for therapeutic strategies to modulate the onset and progression of myocardial and cerebral ischemia.

Potential benefits of PGI_2 and PGE_1 due to their capacity to suppress "pro-inflammatory" events such as platelet aggregation were overlooked because of several in vivo studies in which local administration of prostaglandins of the E series potentiated inflammatory reactions including: vasoactive mediator induced edema (3), C5a (4) and carrageenin (5) induced inflammation. In addition, increases in prostaglandin concentrations at sites of inflammation (6,7) and the suppression of inflammatory reactions by cyclooxygenase inhibitors such as aspirin, indomethacin, and ibuprofen (8,9) suggested that prostaglandins mediated inflammation. The proinflammatory effect of prostaglandins has been ascribed to their ability to cause vasodilation and increase transudation of plasma at sites of inflammation (10,11).

However, several studies beginning in the early 1970's demonstrated the ability of PGE and PGI_2 to suppress the functional response of a variety of inflammatory cells besides platelets. These include mast cells and basophils (12,13), polymorphonuclear leucocytes (14-16), monocytes and macrophages (17), lymphocytes (18), and natural killer cells (19,20). These observations support the hypothesis that PGE and PGI_2 may under certain conditions function as inhibitors of inflammatory reactions. The ability of PGE_1 and PGI_2 to inhibit the functional responses of these inflammatory cells has usually been correlated with their ability to enhance adenylate cyclase activity and increase intracellular cyclic AMP levels. However, a direct cause and effect relationship between the ability of PGE_1 and PGI_2 to inhibit inflammatory cell functional response and induce increased cyclic AMP levels is not definitely established in each cell type.

Several investigators have presented evidence for two mechanisms by which cyclic AMP may modulate inflammatory cell activation. Inhibition of certain platelet aggregation responses by PGE_1 and PGI_2 appears to correlate with the stimulation of a calcium dependent ATPase activity by cyclic AMP (21,22). Stimulation of the enzyme system, located in the dense tubular system, results in sequestration of intracellular calcium and a reduction in stimulus induced increases in intracellular calcium, a process which correlates with impaired cell function. A proposed mechanism by which cyclic AMP may modulate inflammatory cells has been demonstrated in mast cells: Inhibition by PGE of IgE induced mast cell degranulation correlates with increased intracellular cyclic AMP levels, activation of a cyclic AMP dependent protein kinase and subsequent inhibition of the methylation of phosphotidylethanolamine to phosphotidylcholine (23).

Additional studies in neutrophils, platelets, and monocytes suggest that PG may also alter the functional characteristics of specific receptors on cell membranes. Cyclooxygenase products of arachidonic acid metabolism can modulate human platelet fibrinogen receptors (24) and prostacyclin treatment of human platelets inhibits thrombin induced exposure of the receptor for factor VIII von Willibrand factor (25). In addition, prostaglandin treatment of murine macrophages alters expression of Fc and concanavalin A receptors on murine macrophages (26). Neutrophils isolated from rats treated systemically with 15-methyl-PGE_1 (a stable analog of PGE_1) - at concentrations shown to inhibit acute inflammatory reactions in vivo - exhibit decreased generation of superoxide anion production and lysosomal enzyme secretion after stimulation by formyl-methionyl-leucyl-phenylalanine (FMLP) (27). This inhibition of the functional responses of PMN correlates with a two to three fold decrease in the binding affinity of the formyl peptide receptor for its ligand. In these studies there was no consistent alteration in the total number of receptor sites per cell. Recent in vitro studies have confirmed the ability of PGE_1 to alter the binding affinity of PMN formyl peptide receptors. However, it is not known whether changes in receptor binding affinity by PGE_1 are directly related to increases in cyclic AMP levels and/or alteration of phospholipid methylation reactions.

1. MODULATION BY PROSTAGLANDINS OF ACUTE INFLAMMATORY REACTIONS.

1.1 Vasoactive mediator induced vascular permeability: A characteristic series of vascular changes, including an increase in vasopermeability, occur very early in the course of both acute and chronic inflammatory reactions. Increases in vasopermeability and edema formation correlate with occurrence of endothelial cell contraction and gap formation (28). It has been shown (studies described below) that systemic treatment of rats with prostaglandins of the E series inhibits edema formation associated with immune complex induced vasculitis (29), and chronic adjuvant arthritis (30). Therefore it was of interest to examine the roles of systemic prostaglandin treatment on edema formation associated with intradermal challenge with vasoactive mediators. Rats treated systemically with 15-methyl-PGE_1 showed a marked decrease in development of edema formation in skin after local administration of histamine, serotonin, and bradykinin (31). The vasoactive effects of anaphylatoxin C3a and compound 48/80 (an agent which causes mast cell degranulation) were also inhibited by PGE treatment. Suppression of vascular permeability by greater than 80% was observed with either oral or subcutaneous administration of 15-M-PGE_1 and the effect of one dose lasted up to 29 hr after it was given. This is a consequence of the relative resistance of 15-M-PGE_1 to metabolism by 15-prostaglandin-dehydrogenase. The ability of prostaglandins to suppress vascular permeability showed structure specificity since neither PGA_2 nor $PGF_{2\alpha}$ were effective in suppressing permeability responses. The inhibitory activity of PGE_1 on edema formation correlated with a marked decrease in endothelial cell gap formation and preservation of normal endothelial cell junctions. Thus, suppression of vasopermeability by prior systemic PGE treatment may depend on the ability of PGE compounds to preserve the integrity of tight junctions between venule endothelial cells.

1.2 Carrageenin Induced Vascular Permeability Change.

Although local administration of prostaglandin of the E series enhances the acute inflammatory response associated with carrageenin administration in the skin, we have recently examined the effect of systemic PGE_1 treatment on carrageenin induced rat footpad edema. This reaction represents a complex inflammatory system in which there are three distinct phases of mediator induced vascular permeability changes (32). The initial phase during the first 30 min after injection results from release of histamine and serotonin from mast cells and is inhibited by antihistamines. The second phase between 1 and 2.5 hr after injection is attributed to reaction of bradykinin since pretreatment of rats with cellulose sulfate reduces edema. The third phase of persistent edema is complement dependent and has been attributed to local production by inflammatory cells of prostaglandins, especially of the E series. This phase of edema formation is inhibited by indomethacin and aspirin and is potentiated by local injection of vasodilatory prostaglandins such as PGE_2 (33). However, other studies suggest that PGE administration (34) and stimulation of prostaglandin production (35) may reduce carrageenin induced edema formation. Systemic treatment of rats with 15-methyl-PGE_1 exhibits a dose dependent inhibition of all three phases of carrageenin induced edema formation (36). Consistent with the above findings, there is up to a 30% decrease in footpad thickness 1 hr after injection of carrageenin into the footpad. Whereas control animals showed a progressive increase in footpad swelling over the next 5 hr, subcutaneous (systemic) injection of 15-methyl-PGE_1 (1 mg/kg) caused virtually complete suppression of the second and third phases of edema formation. These findings emphasize the marked differences between the local and systemic effect of prostaglandins on acute inflammatory reactions. The ability of PGE_1 to inhibit the later phase of carrageenin induced edema formation, which is in part dependent upon the recruitment of polymorphonuclear leucocytes to the inflammatory site, is consistent with *in vitro* studies demonstrating the ability of PGE to inhibit neutrophil chemotaxis, superoxide anion production, and lysosomal enzyme release. Although PGE_2 concentrations at sites of acute inflammation are increased, it is possible that the delayed permeability changes induced by carrageenin are not secondary to PGE_2 as previously described, but are the result of local production of lipoxygenase products and other secretory products of stimulated neutrophils. Increased PGE levels associated with inflammatory reactions may in fact represent a modulating system that limits the extent of the inflammatory response.

1.3 Immune Complex Induced Tissue Injury

PGE_1 treatment suppresses several immune complex mediated inflammatory reactions including progression of immune complex induced glomerulonephritis in NZB/NZW mice (see below). However, this model of immune complex induced tissue injury represents a complex system in which an inflammatory response and tissue injury develop over a 4 to 5 month period. A cell mediated component has been recognized for full expression of the disease. A more recent study has defined the effects of systemic treatment with PGE_1 on development of immune complex induced vasculitis, the Reverse Passive Arthus reaction (RPA), in the skin of rats. The pathogenesis of the Arthus reaction includes formation of immune complexes in the vessel wall, activation of complement, local generation of chemotactic peptides including C5a, influx of neutrophils in response to the chemotactic products, endocytosis of immune complexes and subsequent release of lysosomal enzymes, superoxide anion, and products of arachidonic acid metabolism resulting in tissue injury. The degree of tissue injury can be quantified readily by the increase in permeability and hemorrhage that develops within 4 hr after deposition of immune complexes.

Systemic treatment of rats with PGE_1 or its stable analog 15-methyl-PGE_1 results in marked suppression of immune complex induced vascular damage in rats (27). Animals treated orally with the stable analog 12 hr before challenge are protected from vascular injury in a dose dependent manner. Immunofluorescence microscopy demonstrates deposition of complement components and the presence of immune complexes in vessel walls, suggesting that PGE_1 treatment does not alter development of the inflammatory response by inhibiting formation of immune complexes and fixation of complement. Studies in vitro show that micromolar concentrations of PGE_1 do not inhibit activation of the complement cascade by soluble immune complexes. However, recruitment of neutrophils from the circulation appears to be inhibited in these animals. Ultrastructural studies demonstrate a paucity of neutrophils in the interstitial compartment and a failure of phagocytosis of immune complexes. Neutrophils harvested from blood of animals treated with PGE_1 or the 15-methyl-PGE_1 analog showed decreased functional responses, including enzyme release and superoxide anion production, following stimulation with chemotactic peptides. Thus the antiinflammatory effects of PGE_1 demonstrated in acute immune complex induced vasculitis experiments appear to be caused in part by interference with functional responsiveness of neutrophils.

In a second model of immune complex mediated tissue injury (the nephrotoxic serum nephritis model), systemic treatment of animals with 15-methyl-PGE_1 suppressed both the glomerular hypercellularity and the proteinuria associated with a single intravenous injection of antibodies directed against rat glomerular basement membrane, without altering binding of specific antibody to the glomerular basement membrane (37). In this model of tissue injury, local activation of complement components and sequestration of polymorphonuclear leucocytes within capillary lumens of glomeruli are thought to be critical to development of tissue injury. These studies provide additional support for the hypothesis that systemic PGE_1 treatment will inhibit immune complex induced inflammatory reactions and that certain prostaglandins may play an important role in regulation of type II immune reactions.

An additional study examining the effects of PGE_1 modulation on the onset and development of a lupus-like glomerulonephritis in specific strains of mice showed that in both NZB/NZW and MRL/1 mice there was increased survival and decreased glomerulonephritis as a result of PGE_1 treatment (38). This inhibitory effect of PGE_1 was associated with a decrease in glomerular deposition of immune complexes. In contrast there is no effect of PGE_1 on either survival or development of glomerular injury in BXSB mice indicating a strain specificity for the immuno modulatory effect of PGE_1. In those strains of mice in which PGE_1 was effective in inhibiting glomerular injury, there was also a significant decrease in circulating levels of the retrovirus envelope glycoprotein gp70 and anti-gp70 antibody immune complexes compared to untreated controls. Since anti-DNA antibody titers were unchanged in PGE_1 treated animals, the data suggest that PGE_1 treatment selectively suppresses the immune response to retroviral gp70. However, both (gp70)-(anti-gp70) and (DNA)-(anti-DNA) immune complex deposition in glomeruli were decreased in PGE_1 treated mice suggesting that PGE_1 treatment may also modulate the effects of additional mediators (i.e. histamine, serotonin, PAF) that may either directly or indirectly influence localization of circulating immune complexes within the glomerular capillary bed. This would be consistent with the previous observations (see above) indicating that PGE_1 treatment suppresses vasoactive mediator induced edema formation.

In another model of immune complex induced glomerulonephritis (induced by daily injection of apoferritin), systemic PGE_1 and PGE_2 treatment resulted in decreased glomerular injury (as monitored by proteinuria) and a change in the pattern of immune complex deposition from a capillalry loop location to the mesangium (39). The protective effect of PGE_1 treatment was dose dependent and correlated with a decrease in circulating anti-apoferritin titers. However, one cannot rule out the possibility that PGE_1 inhibition of immune complex mediated glomerular injury was secondary to alternative mechanisms such as those mentioned above.

Further evidence for the ability of prostaglandins to modulate vascular injury and edema formation is provided by studies examining the effects of these agents on development of Passive Cutaneous Anaphylaxis in rabbits (40). PGE_1 administered intravenously inhibited transudation of proteins in the skin of rabbits at sites of initiation of the anaphylactic response. This inhibition of Passive Cutaneous Anaphylactic reactions in rabbits was observed with other pharmacologic agents that are known to increase intracellular levels of cyclic AMP. These studies suggest that PGE_1 may modulate acute inflammatory reactions by increasing levels of cAMP in inflammatory cells. This would include inhibition of platelet aggregation as well as modulation of mast cell degranulation.

1.4 Effects of Prostaglandins on Intravascular Phlogistic Agents.

Systemic treatment of rabbits with PGI_2 inhibits the neutropenia and thrombocytopenia associated with subsequent infusion of immune complexes (41). PGI_2 did not alter the interaction of immune complexes with polymorphonuclear membrane receptors in vitro but did inhibit aggregation and secretion of platelet activating factor (PAF) induced by immune complexes. In a separate study, intravenous infusion of prostacyclin (10-50 ng/kg/min) in rabbits inhibited PAF induced neutropenia, thrombocytopenia and sequestration of polymorphonuclears in the pulmonary capillary bed (42). These observations support the hypothesis that PGI_2 has antiinflammatory activity and suggest a physiologic role for PGI_2 in modulating the interaction between immune complexes and neutrophils. Additional studies in mongrel dogs indicate that prostacyclin infusion inhibits an increase in filtration coefficient and in lung vascular permeability changes following microembolization (43). Since microembolization in the lung is associated with acute lung injury and is dependent on the presence of circulating neutrophils (44), the data support the view that PGI_2 may be an important regulator of neutrophil activation within the vascular compartment. In addition the data support previous observations implicating PGI_2 as an important modulator of vascular tone and suggest a critical role for PGI_2 in development of acute pulmonary hypertension.

Systemic prostacyclin treatment prolongs survival and inhibits pulmonary vascular changes associated with intravenous infusion of endotoxin (45). Endotoxin mediated lung injury depends upon neutrophil and platelet activation as well as activation of the clotting system and fibrin deposition. After infusion of PGI_2 there is not only an improvement in the pulmonary hemodynamic parameters associated with endotoxin administration, there is also an increase in numbers of circulating platelets and a decrease in fibrin degradation products. In view of these observations, it is of interest that intravascular infusion of prostacyclin reduces some of the clinical changes associated with pulmonary embolism (43). Although the mechanisms whereby PGI_2 inhibit the tissue injury associated with endotoxemia are not clear, several are possible including inhibition of platelet aggregation, inhibition of neutrophil functional responses, and vasodilation. Similar findings were observed in rats in that intravenous infusion of prostacyclin inhibited development of the generalized Schwartzman reaction (46). Infusion of prostacyclin to a mean dose of 57 ng/kg/min before and after administration of endotoxin inhibited development of fibrin and platelet thrombi within capillaries. There was also an attenuation of endotoxin induced decreases in renal blood flow and glomerular filtration. Prostacyclin treatment also inhibited completely the endotoxin induced decrease in circulating platelet counts.

1.5 Effects of Prostaglandins on Bronchoconstriction.

As mentioned previously both PGI_2 and prostaglandins of the E series have potent vasodilatory activities (10,11). This has prompted interest in the possibility that the smooth muscle relaxant effects of these agents might extend to the airways, implicating PGI_2 and PGE as potentially important bronchodilator agents. Several reports indicate that PGI_2 attenuates bronchoconstriction induced by $PGF_{2\alpha}$ in dogs (47), inhibits histamine induced bronchospasm in guinea pigs (48) and 5-hydroxytryptamine (5-HT) induced bronchoconstriction in mongrel cats (49). These latter studies indicate that bolus intravenous administration of PGI_2 in microgram quantities to cats will reverse 5-HT induced bronchoconstriction and suggest that PGI_2 and PGE may function as endogenous regulators of bronchial muscle tone and possibly serve as potential therapeutic agents in asthma patients.

However, application of PGI_2 as a therapeutic agent in the treatment of asthmatic patients is not defined. An initial study indicates that PGI_2 prevents a specifically induced bronchoconstriction in asthmatic patients (50) whereas a second study failed to show consistent changes in pulmonary function in asthmatic patients following PGI_2 administration (51). Additional studies have shown that PGE_1 in a lipid emulsion inhibits both the onset and severity of bronchoconstriction induced by aerosol administration of histamine in guinea pigs (48). This inhibitory activity of PGE_1 correlates with its bronchodilator effects.

2. REGULATION BY PROSTAGLANDINS OF EXPERIMENTAL MODELS OF CHRONIC INFLAMMATION

Metabolites of arachidonic acid are known to play a key role in the regulation of diverse physiological systems. A prime example of the modulator effect of these ubiquitous fatty acids is their ability to regulate the function of cells which participate in acute inflammatory reactions. In addition, inflammatory cells associated with more long-lived, chronic immune reactions also are influenced by products of arachidonic acid metabolism. A number of reports describe the immunomodulating role of arachidonic acid metabolites (52,53). Here, we examine the ability of separate arachidonic acid metabolites to influence development and progression of several chronic immune reactions.

2.1 Modulation by Prostaglandins of Lymphocyte and Macrophage Functions In Vitro.

Before discussing the effects of prostaglandins on animal models of inflammation, it might be useful to outline the ability of certain arachidonic acid metabolites to regulate lymphocyte and macrophage function, since these cells are crucial to development of chronic immune responses. Current experimental evidence indicates that addition of arachidonic acid products profoundly influences lymphocyte transformation (53), cell mediated cytotoxicity (54), and production of soluble mediators involved in the initiation and maintenance of cell mediated immune responses. With regard to production of inflammatory mediators, Gordon et. al. (55) and Bray et. al. (56) demonstrated that prostaglandins of the E series suppress lymphokine production, as monitored by macrophage migration inhibition. More recently, Rappaport and Dodge (57) and Baker et. al. (58) have demonstrated that exogenous PGE inhibits another lymphocyte product, interleukin 2 (Il-2). PGE was the only classical prostaglandin shown to suppress Il-2 production, as PGF and PGA were both ineffective. Cyclooxygenase inhibitors increased production of Il-2 above normal levels, supporting the view that endogenous PGE might modulate production of Il-2. Since lymphocyte products are intimately associated with macrophage activation and initiation of cell mediated immune mechanisms, regulation of these lymphocyte-derived mediators might be an important way to regulate chronic inflammation.

Several arachidonic acid metabolites have also been associated with modulation of macrophage activation and subsequent expression and/or release of macrophage-derived products. Snyder et. al. (59) have suggested that prostaglandins can regulate lymphokine induced expression of I-region associated (Ia) antigens or macrophages. Both PGE_1 and PGE_2 (10^{-9} - 10^{-10} M) reduced by 50% the number of Ia positive macrophages normally induced by conditioned T-cell media. Addition of thromboxane B_2 antagonized the effect of PGE compounds. The stable analog of PGE_1, 15-methyl-PGE_1, can influence lymhokine-dependent reexpression of Ia antigens by cultured macrophages isolated from pulmonary granulomas (60). As shown in Fig. 1, 6 x 10^{-7} M 15-methyl-PGE completely suppressed the ability of lymphokine stimulated, cultured granuloma macrophages to reexpress Ia antigen throughout the entire study period. The same concentration of $PGF_{2\alpha}$ failed to influence reexpression of Ia antigen. Similarly, Steeg et. al. (61) demonstrated that partially purified gamma interferon could induce cultured P388D cell line macrophages and thioglycollate-elicited peritoneal macrophages to express Ia antigen and that this expression could be abrogated in a dose dependent manner by 10^{-10} to 10^{-6} M PGE_2. Whereas PGE compounds suppress macrophage Ia antigen expression, a preliminary study indicates that lipoxygenase products, especially the monohydroxyeicosatetraenoic acids, may potentiate the expression of Ia antigens by macrophages in the presence of lymphokine (60). In addition to regulation of Ia antigen expression by macrophages, PGE has been implicated in the regulation of lymphocyte-activating factor/interleukin (Il-1) production (62). By no means is Il-1 the only macrophage-derived product that is regulated by PGE, since this autocoid appears to dictate the production of complement proteins (63), plasminogen activator (64) and lysosomal hydrolase (65) by various macrophage populations. Through in vitro studies such as those discussed above, the ability of prostaglandins to "down-regulate" specific inflammatory cell functions can be examined. With the introduction of unique animal models, these studies can be expanded in order to study in vivo the regulation of immune cell reactivity and alterations in host defenses.

2.2 Experimental Animal Models.

2.2.1 Adjuvant-induced polyarthritis. Early studies by Aspinall and Cammarata (66) provided some of the first evidence that PGE_2 could be

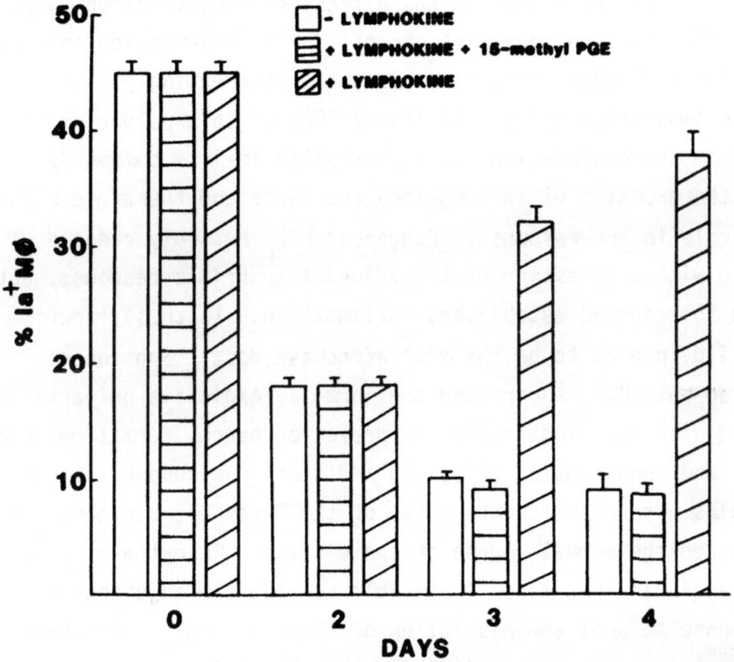

Figure 1. Effect of 15-methyl-PGE_1 on re-expression of Ia antigen *in vitro* by granuloma macrophages. At day zero, the percentages of Ia positive macrophages isolated from Schistosome egg-induced granulomatous lesions was approximately 4570. Lymphokine, isolated from lymphocytes sensitized to the Schistosome antigen, treated induced a re-expression of Ia, which was suppressed by 5×10^{-7} 15-methyl-PGE_1.

effective as both a prophylactic and therapeutic agent in the modulation of an inflammatory response. In these studies the effects of PGE_2 treatment were examined on the development and course of chronic joint inflammation induced by a single injection of Freunds complete adjuvant. Interestingly, the incentive to examine the immunoregulating activity of PGE_2 on this polyarthritic response stemmed from the observations that prostaglandin-like compounds were commonly found in the exudates of inflammatory reactions and therefore might have a modulating role in the response. Exogenous PGE_2 not only reduced swelling associated with progression of the adjuvant arthritis response, but was also effective in reducing established inflammation. In these experiments 500 μg of PGE_2 (b.i.d) proved to be the most effective dose. Subsequent studies demonstrated that PGE_1 suppressed the normally explosive polyarthritis response associated with this model (30) and prevented pannus formation, cartilage degradation and bone erosion (67). In addition, the suppressive effect of the prostaglandins was restricted to those of the E series, since neither $PGF_{2\alpha}$ nor PGA_2 altered the normal course of the disease. Recent availability of stable prostaglandin analogs made it possible to test the adjuvant-induced polyarthritic response to oral administration of 15-methyl-PGE_1. As shown in Fig. 2, the inflammatory response was inhibited by the orally active 15-methyl PGE_1 in a dose dependent manner. As little as 50 μg 15-methyl-PGE_1, given once a day during the study period, was effective. The histopathological changes characteristic of an inflamed synovium, including an inflammatory cell infiltrate and pannus formation, were suppressed by varying degrees at each dose studied. The activity and stability of orally administered 15-methyl-PGE_1 probably lies in the protection of the hydroxyl group at the 15-position, since suppression of inflammation was not observed in animals treated orally with PGE_1, PGE_2, PGI_2 or 16,16 dimethyl PGE_1.

2.2.2 NZB/NZW and MRL/1 murine models of systemic lupus erythematosus. The study of the autoimmune disease systemic lupus erythematosus (SLE) has been advanced through use of two murine strains that develop a lupus-like disorder. The F_1 hybrid of New Zealand black and New Zealand white mice (NZB/W) and the MRL/1 mouse both develop a chronic, autoimmune disease characterized by the appearance of autoantibodies that leads to a fatal nephritis. A single 200 μg injection of PGE_1, given daily, prevents the clinical glomerulonephritis associated with this syndrome (68). Although autoantibodies to nuclear antigens were not suppressed, the survival rate among NZB/W mice was enhanced during the one year study period. Renal mor-

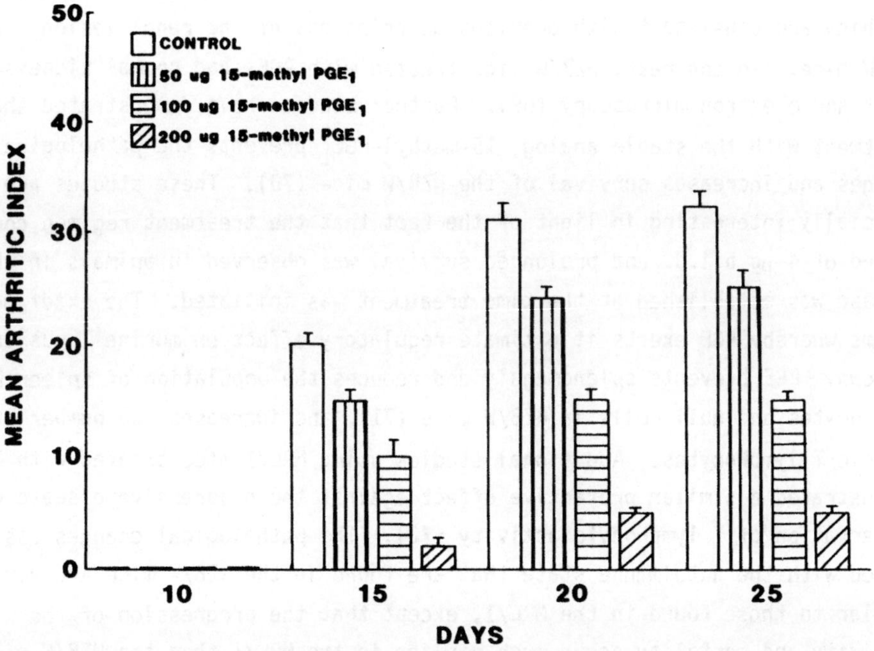

Figure 2. Effect of 15-methyl-PGE$_1$ on development of adjuvant polyarthritis. Prostaglandin was given orally once each day from time of adjuvant challenge. Time is expressed as days post adjuvant challenge.

phology of untreated animals at 58-65 weeks demonstrated enlarged glomeruli with marked proliferation of cells and thickening of basement membranes, all of which are consistent with previous descriptions of the renal lesions in NZB/W mice. In contrast, NZB/W mice treated with PGE_1 had normal kidneys by light and electron microscopy (69). Further studies have demonstrated that treatment with the stable analog, 15-methyl-PGE_1 prevents the pathological changes and increases survival of the NZB/W mice (70). These studies are especially interesting in light of the fact that the treatment regimen consisted of 4 μg b.i.d. and prolonged survival was observed in animals in whom disease was established at the time treatment was initiated. The exact mechanisms whereby PGE exerts it ultimate regulatory effect on murine lupus are unknown. PGE prevents splenomegaly and reduces the population of spleen B lymphocytes and null cells in NZB/W mice (71), and increases the number of splenic T lymphocytes. Additional studies using MRL/1 mice treated with PGE_1 demonstrated a similar protective effect against the progressive disease with preservation of T lymphocyte activity (72). The pathological changes associated with the autoimmune state that are found in the NZB/W mice are very similar to those found in the MRL/1, except that the progression of the morbidity and mortality occur much earlier in the MRL/1 than the NZB/W mice. This observation may explain why neither PGE_1 nor 15-methyl-PGE_1 had a suppressive effect on MRL/1 mice with established nephritis (73). As noted, the beneficial effects of systemic 15-methyl-PGE_1 were documented in an additional animal model of nephritis, nephrotoxic serum nephritis (37). Proteinuria and glomerular hypercellularity normally associated with this disease were significantly suppressed in a dose dependent manner by the PGE_1 analog. Nonetheless, deposition of antibody in the glomerular basement membrane (characteristic of this disease state) was not altered.

2.2.3 Hypersensitivity and foreign body-type granulomatous inflammation. We have examined the effect of systemically administered prostaglandins on development of hypersensitivity and foreign body-type granulomas in mice (74). Foreign body-type granulomas were induced in mice by the embolization of Sephadex beads, while the hypersensitivity or immune granuloma was generated by the embolization of *Schistosoma mansoni* eggs. The hypersensitivity granuloma is a well established model of cell mediated immune reactions, whose development and modulation involve helper/effector and suppressor T lymphocyte subsets (75). By employing these models and allowing granulomas to develop in a synchronous phase, we could easily examine the immunoregulating role of several arachidonic acid metabolites on initiation, maintenance, and resolution of the chronic lesions. As shown in Table I, the granuloma size around embolized Schistosome eggs increased linearly over the 16 day study period. In 15-methyl-PGE_1 treated animals hypersensitivity granulomas were dramatically suppressed, reaching a mean area by day 16 post-challenge of only 30% that of the control. In contrast, immune granuloma development in PGF_2 treated animals was augmented at day 4 and 8 post-challenge by 60% and 39%, respectively. At day 16, the granuloma areas were not significantly different from those of saline treated controls. The most striking evidence that the two prostaglandins were manipulating an immune component of the hypersensitivity lesion stemmed from studies examining development of foreign body-type granuloma in the treated mice. Neither 15-methyl-PGE_1 nor $PGF_{2\alpha}$ affected the proliferative response of the granuloma to the less immunogenic polysaccharide bead, Sephadex (Table I). The above observation, that the hypersensitivity-type granuloma lesion was suppressed while the nonspecific foreign body granuloma was not, is most likely related to a difference in the degree of lymphocyte involvement. The hypersensitivity lesion is a response to a natural granuloma-inducing nidus that results in highly active T cells, while the response to the foreign body granuloma lacks specific T lymphocyte sensitization. In the hypersensitivity granuloma as in all cell mediated immune responses, lymphocytes are necessary (76). Thus, it was important to examine available lymphoid tissue, (splenic tissue) for prostaglandin-induced alterations in lymphocyte numbers and function. As the normal hypersensitivity lung lesions developed over the 16 day study period, total spleen cells increased; actual numbers were found to increase by 30×10^6 cells by day 16 post-challenge. In contrast, splenic lymphocytes did not increase in 15-methyl-PGE_1 treated animals. $PGF_{2\alpha}$ treatment caused an increase in numbers of splenic lymphocytes at day 8, followed by a reduction in total lymphocytes at day 16. The percentage of splenic T and B lymphocytes were also examined. In control animals, the percentage of T lymphocytes remained constant over the 16 day study period, while B lymphocytes increased modestly. In those animals treated with $PGF_{2\alpha}$, a general decrease in total T lymphocytes was found, while the B cell percentage increased. However, PGE_1 treatment caused a dramatic decrease in B lymphocytes, while total T lymhocytes increased. These observations are similar to those made in NZB/W mice treated with PGE (71). In an effort to examine the means whereby prostaglandins modulate development of the granuloma, a series of lymphocyte sensitization/transfer experiments were performed. Experiments were designed to determine whether prostaglandin treatment affected granuloma development via the induction or elicitation arm of the immune sysem: Spleen cells from donor mice sensitized by Schistosome egg challenge were adoptively transferred to naive mice, pulmonary granulomas induced, and the animals treated with 15-methyl-PGE_1. As shown in Table II, the adoptively transferred, sensitized lymphocytes did enhance the normal granulomatous response, whereas the response in the 15-methyl-PGE_1 treated animals was suppressed. Prostaglandin treatment was also shown to influence induction of immunoreactive lymphocytes: In this study spleen cells recovered from mice that received Schistosome eggs and prostaglandin treatment were transferred to normal mice and examined for their ability to alter the normal development of the granuloma. As previously observed, spleen cells from the untreated sensitized donor gave an enhanced inflammatory response, whereas spleen cells from 15-methyl-PGE_1 treated donors significantly suppressed the ability to adoptively transfer this delayed-type hypersensitivity response (Table II). To further investigate the mechanism by which the prostaglandins exert their immunoregulating influence, we studied the *in vivo* kinetics of Ia antigen expression by granulomatous macrophages isolated from synchronous pulmonary lesions in treated and untreated animals. As shown in Fig. 3, the percentage of granuloma macrophages isolated from control mice expressing Ia antigen increased significantly during the 16 day study period. Animals receiving exogenous $PGF_{2\alpha}$ demonstrated an increase in the percentage of granuloma macrophages expressing Ia antigen when examined during the early development of the granuloma. The percentage of Ia antigen positive granuloma macrophages were shown to increase by 46% at day 4 and 24% at day 8 post-challenge. In contrast, the expression of Ia antigen by granuloma macrophages isolated from 15-methyl-PGE_1 treated animals was suppressed by approximately 70% (Fig. 3). This paralleled the cellular infiltrate observed as the synchronous lesions developed in animals on various treatment protocols. The suppression of Ia antigen-bearing granuloma macrophages by exogenous 15-methyl-PGE_1 was found to be dose dependent, with as little as 15 μg/kg resulting in suppression of Ia antigen (9). Since PGE acts therapeutically in rats with established adjuvant arthritis and in NZB/W mice with established nephritis, it was of interest to assess the effect of 15-methyl-PGE on *preformed* hypersensitivity lesions. Pulmonary granulomas were allowed to develop in mice for 8 days before prostaglandin therapy was initiated. This protocol allowed for vigorous development of the immune response before

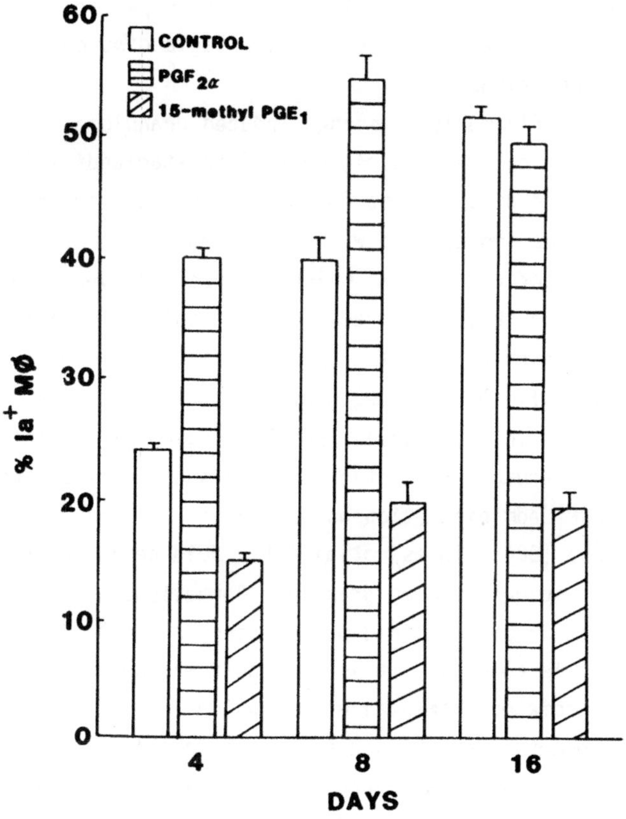

Figure 3. Effect of 15-methyl-PGE$_1$ and PGF$_{2\alpha}$ on the kinetics of Ia antigen expression by granuloma macrophages isolated from synchronously developing lesions. Animals received 1.5 mg/kg prostaglandin from day of challenge.

treatment. As demonstrated in Table III, 15-methyl-PGE_1 treatment resulted in an involution of the normal response. In addition, the percentage of Ia antigen positive granuloma macrophages isolated from these animals was significantly suppressed, reaching a mean of only 30% of the control value at day 16. Treatment with $PGF_{2\alpha}$ did not result in a significant therapeutic effect. These observations demonstrate that certain prostaglandins can arrest ongoing cell mediated immune reactions.

Another model of chronic inflammation - sponge induced granuloma formation - has been used to determine the possible role of prostaglandins in chronic inflammation. Inhibition of granuloma formation was observed when carrageenan-injected sponges were impregnated with large amounts of PGE_2 (77). In essential fatty acid deficient rats, which produce only very small amounts of prostaglandins because they lack precursors, granuloma formation is enhanced (78). The increased chronic inflammatory response is associated with increased collagen synthesis (79). Thus, endogenous prostaglandins might act to suppress chronic inflammation in this model. PGE_1 injection (1 μg/sponge) upon implantation enhanced the acute inflammation and the subsequent production of granuloma, whereas PGE_1 administration on days 4 to 7 inhibited subsequent growth of granuloma (80). In essential fatty acid deficient rats as little as 0.05 μg PGE_1 per sponge reduced granuloma formation.

It is clear that the role of phospholipid metabolites in regulation of immune/inflammatory reactions is complex. It is not known why PGE should have an effect on inflammation in some experimental models which is similar to compounds (e.g., aspirin and indomethacin) which are able to inhibit prostaglandin synthesis. But then, it is not absolutely clear how the traditional nonsteroidal antiinflammatory agents work. It does appear that inhibition of cyclooxygenase activity is important to their effect, but they do not inhibit lipoxygenase activity the products of which are also mediators of inflammation. Thus the paradox remains. How it will be resolved is unknown, but the search for the answers promises to be fascinating.

Table 1. Effect of 15-methyl PGE_1 and $PGE_{2\alpha}$ on the proliferative response induced by hypersensitivity or foreign body-type granulomas. Animals received 1.5 mg/kg of prostaglandin from day of challenge.

	Immune Granuloma (mean area x 10^{-3} μm^{-2})			Foreign Body Granuloma (mean area x 10^{-3} μm^{-2})		
	DAYS	POST	CHALLENGE	DAYS	POST	CHALLENGE
Treatment	4.0	8.0	16.0	4.0	8.0	16.0
15-methyl PGE_1	9.6	19.8	40.0	--	8.2	--
$PGF_{2\alpha}$	15.9	28.4	44.8	--	6.9	--
Control	6.4	10.2	11.8	--	7.5	--

Table 2. Effect of 15-methyl PGE_1 on induction (A) and elicitation (B) of the hypersensitivity granulomatous response. Animals were given 1.5 mg/kg/day 15-methyl PGE_1. For the elicitation study 3 x 10^7 spleen cells were adaptively transferred, while 5 x 10^7 spleen cells were used in the induction study.

Recipient treatment	Donor treatment	Activity of transferred cells	Granuloma Area (x 10^{-3} μm^{-2})
A. --	Saline	Normal	22
--	Saline	Sensitized	44
--	15-methyl PGE_1	Sensitized	26
B. Saline	--	Normal	22
Saline	--	Sensitized	38
15-methyl PGE_1	--	Sensitized	15

Table 3. Therapeutic effect of 15-methyl PGE_1: Reduction of granuloma size and Ia antigen expression in preformed lesions. Granulomas were allowed to develop for 8 days prior to 15-methyl PGE_1 treatment (animals were given 1.5 mg/kg from day 8 to day 16).

	Granuloma Area (x 10^{-3} μm^{-2})			Ia+ Granuloma MO (Percent)		
	DAYS	POST	CHALLENGE	DAYS	POST	CHALLENGE
Treatment	4.0	8.0	16.0	4.0	8.0	16.0
Control	9.5	22.0	41.1	22.1	45.2	52.2
15-methyl PGE_1	9.6	22.0	20.1	22.1	45.2	20.4

REFERENCES

1. Kloeze J: Influence of prostaglandins on platelet adhesiveness and platelet aggregation. Prostaglandins, Proceeding of the II Nobel Symposium, 1966. ed. S. Bergstrom and B. Samuelsson. London. Interscience 1967, p. 271-278.
2. Smith JB: The prostanoids in hemostasis and thrombosis, a review. Am J Pathol (99):740-805, 1980.
3. Williams TJ, Morley J: Prostaglandins as potentiators of increased vascular permeability in inflammation. Nature (256):215-217, 1973.
4. Wedmore CV, Williams TJ: Control of vascular permeability by polymorphonuclear leucocytes in inflammation. Nature (289):646-650, 1981.
5. Williams TJ, Peck MJ: Role of prostaglandin-mediated vasodilatation in inflammation. Nature (270):530-532, 1977.
6. Thomas G: Characteristics of prostaglandin E_1 potentiation of inflammatory activity of some agents. Prostaglandins (19):39-50, 1980.
7. Thomas G, West GB: Prostaglandins, kinin and inflammation in the rat. Br J Pharmacol (50):231-235, 1974.
8. Jones SA, Kennedy AJ, Roberts NA: Assessment of drugs for activity in established Type II collagen arthritis. Agents Actions (12):650-656, 1982.
9. Bailey PJ, Strum A: Immune complexes and inflammation. A study of the activity of antiinflammatory drugs in the Reverse Passive Arthus Reaction. Biochem Pharm (32):475-481, 1983.
10. Grennan DM, Mitchel W, Miller W, Zeitlin IJ: The effects of prostaglandin E_1, bradykinin and histamine on canine synovial vascular permeability. Br J Pharmacol (60):251-258, 1977.
11. Echt M, Gauer OH, Kapteina F, Lang L: Effects of prostaglandin E_2 and $F_{2\alpha}$ on cutaneous arteries and veins *in vivo* in the isolated rabbit ear. *In*: Bergstrom S (ed) Advances in the Biosciences, 9th International Conference on Prostaglandins. Pergamon Press, Oxford, 1978, p 353.
12. Lichtenstein LM, DiBarnardo R: The immediate allergic response: *in vitro* action of cyclic AMP and other drugs on the two stages of histamine release. J Immunol (107):1131-1137, 1971.
13. Foreman JC, Hallett MD, Mongard JL: The relationship between histamine secretion and ^{45}calcium uptake by mast cells. J Physiol (271):193-202, 1977.
14. Rivkin I, Rosenblatt J, Becker EL: The role of cyclic AMP in the chemotactic responsiveness and spontaneous motility of rabbit peritoneal neutrophils. J Immunol (115):1126-1134, 1975.
15. Zurier RB, Weissmann G, Hoffstein S, Kammerman S, Tai HH: Mechanisms of lysosomal enzyme release from human leucocytes. J Clin Invest (53):297-309. 1974.
16. Marone G, Thomas LL, Lichtenstein LM: The role of agonists that activate adenylate cyclase in the control of cAMP metabolism and enzyme release by human polymorphonuclear leucocytes. J Immunol (125):2277-2283, 1980.
17. Lehmeyer JE, Johnston RB Jr: Effect of antiinflammatory drugs and agents that elevate intracellular cyclic AMP on the release of toxic oxygen metabolites by phagocytes: Studies in a model of tissue-bound IgG. Clin Immunol Immunopathol (9):482-490, 1978.
18. Goodwin JS, Kaszubowski PA, Williams RC: Cyclic adenosine monophosphate response to prostaglandin E_2 on subpopulations of human lymphocytes. J Exp Med (150):1260-1264, 1979.

19. Katz P, Zaytoun AM, Fauci AJ: Mechanisms of cell mediated cytotoxicity. I. Modulation of natural killer cell activity by cyclic nucleotides. J Immunol (129):287-296, 1982.
20. Goto T, Herberman RB, Maluish A, Strong DM: Cyclic AMP as a mediator of prostaglandin E-induced suppression of human natural killer cell activity. J Immunol (130):1350-1355, 1983.
21. Kaser-Glanzmann L, Jakabova M, George JN, Luscher EF: Stimulation of calcium uptake in platelet membrane vesicles by adenosine 3',5'-cyclic monophosphase and protein kinase. Biochem Biophys Acta (466):429-446, 1977.
22. Cutler L, Rodnan GP, Feinstein MD: Cytochemical localization of adenylate cyclase and of calcium ion, magnesium ion activated ATPase in the dense tubular system of human blood platelets. Biochim Biophys Acta (542):357-365, 1978.
23. Hirata F, Axelrod J: Phospholipid methylation and biological signal transmission. Science (209):1082-1090, 1980.
24. Morinelli TA, Niewiarowski S, Kornecki E, Figures WR, Wachtfogel Y, Colman RW: Platelet aggregation and exposure of fibrinogen receptors by prostaglandin endoperoxide analogues. Blood (61):41-49, 1983.
25. Fujimota T, Ohara S, Hawiger J: Thrombin induced exposure and prostacyclin inhibition of the receptor for factor VII/von Willebrand Factor on human platelets. J Clin Invest (69):1212-1219, 1982.
26. Razin E, Globerson A: The effect of various prostaglandins on plasma membrane receptors and function of mouse macrophages. Adv Exp Med Biol (114):415-419, 1979.
27. Fantone JC, Marasco WA, Elgas LJ, Ward PA: Modulation of rat neutrophil function in vivo by prostaglandins. J Immunol (130):1495-1497, 1983.
28. Cotran RS, Majno G: A light and electron microscopic analysis of vascular injury. Ann NY Acad Sci (116):750-765, 1964.
29. Kunkel SL, Thrall RS, McCormick JR, Ward PA, Zurier RB: Suppression of immune complex vasculitis in rats by prostaglandins. J Clin Invest (64):1525-1529, 1979.
30. Zurier RB, Quagliata F: Effects of prostaglandin E_1 on adjuvant arthritis. Nature (234):304-305, 1971.
31. Fantone JC, Kunkel SL, Ward PA, Zurier RB: Suppression by prostaglandin E_1 of vascular permeability induced by vasoactive mediators. J Immunol (125):2591-2595, 1980.
32. DiRosa M, Groud JP, Willoughby DA: Studies of the mediators of the acute inflammatory response induced in rats in different sites by carrageenin and turpentine. J Pathol (104):15-29, 1971.
33. Bonta IL, Parnham MJ: Time dependent stimulatory and inhibitory effects of prostaglandin E_1 on exudative and tissue components of granulomatous inflammation in rats. Br J Pharmacol (65):465-572, 1975.
34. Zurier RB, Hoffstein S, Weissmann G: Suppression of acute and chronic inflammation in adrenalectomized rats by pharmacologic amounts of prostaglandins. Arthritis Rheum (16):606-617, 1973.
35. Robak J, Trakka EK, Daniel Z: The influence of three prostaglandin biosynthesis stimulators on carrageenin induced edema of rat paw. Biochem Pharm (29):1863-1866, 1980.
36. Fantone JC, Kunkel SL, Weingarten B: Inhibition of carrageenin-induced rat footpad edema by systemic treatment with prostaglandins of the E series. Biochem Pharmacol (31):3126-3128, 1982.
37. Kunkel SL, Zanetti M, Sapin C: Suppression of nephrotoxic serum nephritis in rats by prostaglandins E_1. Am J Pathol (108):240-245, 1982.

38. Izui S, Kelley VE, McConahey PJ, Dixon FJ: Selective suppression of retroviral gp70-anti gp70 immune complex formation by prostaglandin E_1 in murine systemic lupus erythematosus. J Exp Med (152):1654-1658, 1980.
39. McLeish KR, Gohara AF, Stelzer GT, Wallace JH: Treatment of murine immune complex glomerulonephritis with prostaglandin E_2: Dose-response of immune complex deposition, antibody synthesis, and glomerular damage. Clin Immunol Immunopathol (26):18-23, 1983.
40. Kravis T, Zvaifler N: Alteration of rabbit PCA reaction by drugs known to influence intracellular cyclic AMP. J Immunol (113):244-250, 1974.
41. Camussi G, Bussolino F, Tetta C, Caligariscappio F, Coda R, Macchiorlatti E, Alberton M, Roffinello C, Segoloni G: Effect of prostacyclin (PGI_2) on immune-complex-induced neutropenia. Immunology (48):625-633, 1983.
42. Camussi G, Tetta C, Bussolino F: Inhibitory effect of prostacyclin (PGI_2) on neutropenia induced by intravenous injection of platelet-activating-factor (PAF) in the rabbit. Prostaglandins (25):343-351, 1983.
43. Hirose T, Aoki E, Domae M, Masayoshi I, Ikeda T, Tanaka K: The effect of prostacyclin infusion on increased pulmonary vascular permeability following microembolization in dogs. Prostaglandins Leukotrienes Med (11):51-61, 1983.
44. Johnson A, Malik AB: Pulmonary edema after glass bead microembolization: Protective effect of granulocytopenia. J Appl Phys Resp Environ Exer Phys (52):155-163, 1982.
45. Fletcher JR, Ramwell PW: The effects of prostacyclin (PGI_2) on endotoxin shock and endotoxin-induced platelet aggregation in dogs. Circ Shock (7):299-308, 1980.
46. Campo A, Kim Y, Azar SH, Vernier RL, Michael AF: Prevention of the generalized Schwartzman reaction in pregnant rats by prostacyclin infusion. Lab Invest (48):705-710, 1983.
47. Wasserman MA, Cucharma DW, Griffin RL, Wendling MG, DeGrof GL: Bronchial and cardiovascular actions of prostacyclin (PGI_2). Pharmacologist (19):145, 1975 (abst).
48. Mizushima Y, Hishi K, Aihara H, Kurachi M: Inhibition of bronchoconstriction by aerosol of a lipid emulsion containing prostaglandin E_1. J Pharm Pharmacol (35):397, 1983.
49. Spannhake EW, Levin JL, Mellion BT, Gruetter CA, Hyman AL, Kadowitz PJ: Reversal of 5 HT-induced bronchoconstriction by PGI_2: distribution of central and peripheral actions. J Appl Physiol (49):521-527, 1980.
50. Blanco SM, Robuschi M, Ceserani R, Gandolfi C, Kanburoff PJ: Prevention of a specifically induced bronchoconstriction by PGI_2 and 10-methyl-PGI_2 in asthmatic patients. Pharmacol Res Commun (10):657-674, 1978.
51. Szczeklik A, Gryglewski RI, Nizankowski E, Nizankowski R, Musial J: Pulmonary and anti-platelet effects of intravenous and inhaled prostacyclin in man. Prostaglandins (11):651-660, 1978.
52. Goodwin JS, Webb DR: Regulation of immune responses by prostaglandins. Clin Immunol Immunopathol (15):106-113, 1980.
53. Kunkel SL, chensue SW: Prostaglandins and the regulation of immune responses. Adv Inflamm Res (7):93-109, 1983.
54. Henney CS, Bourne HR, Lichtenstein LM: The role of cyclic AMP in the specific cytolytic activity of lymphocytes. J Immunol (108):1526-1534, 1971.
55. Gordon D, Bray MA, Morley J: Control of lymphokine secretion by prostaglandins. Nature (262):401-402, 1976.

56. Bray MA, Gordon D, Morley J: Prostaglandins as regulators in cellular immunity. Prostaglandin Med (1):183-190, 1978.
57. Rappaport RS, Dodge GR: Prostaglandin E inhibits the production of human interleukin 2. J Exp Med (155):943-948, 1982.
58. Baker PE, Fahey JV, Munck A: Prostaglandin inhibition of T cell proliferation is mediated at two levels. Cell Immunol (61):52-60, 1981.
59. Snyder DS, Beller DI, Unanue ER: Prostaglandins modulate macrophage Ia expression. Nature (299):163-165, 1982.
60. Kunkel SL, Chensue SW, Plewa M, Higashi G: Macrophage function in the Schistosoma mansoni egg-induced pulmonary granuloma. Role of arachidonic acid metabolites in macrophage Ia antigen expression. Am J Pathol (114):240-249, 1984.
61. Steeg PS, Johnson HM, Oppenheim J: Regulation of murine macrophage Ia antigen expression by an immune interferon-like lymphokine: Inhibitory effect of endotoxin. J Immunol (129):2402-2406, 1982.
62. Dinarello CA, Marnoy SO, Rosenwasser LJ: Role of arachidonate metabolism in the immunoregulatory function of human leucocytic pyrogen/lymphocyte-activating factor/interleukin 1. J Immunol (130):890-895, 1983.
63. Rediske JJ, Pickering RJ: Arachidonic acid and serum-opsonized zymosan-mediated inhibition of complement production by macrophages. Cell Immunol (in press).
64. Vassalli JD, Hamilton J, Reich E: Macrophage plasminogen activator: modulation of enzyme production by antiinflammatory steroids, mediator inhibitors, and cyclic nucleotides. Cell (8):271-281, 1976.
65. Zurier RB, Dukor P, Weissmann G: Effect of cyclic AMP and colchicine on hydrolase releases from phagocytes. Clin Res (19):453, 1971.
66. Aspinall RL, Cammarata PS: Effect of prostaglandin E_2 on adjuvant arthritis. Nature (224):1320-1321, 1969.
67. Zurier RB, Ballas M: Prostaglandin E_1 suppression of adjuvant arthritis. Histopathology. Arthritis Rheum (16):251-258, 1973.
68. Zurier RB, Sayadoff DM, Torrey SB, Rothfield NR: Prostaglandin E_1 treatment of NZB/NZW mice. I. Prolonged survival of female mice. Arthritis Rheum (20):723-728, 1977.
69. Zurier RB, Damjanov I, Sayadoff DM, Rothfield NR: Prostaglandin E_1 treatment of NZB/NZW E_1 hybrid mice. II. Prevention of glomerulonephritis. Arthritis Rheum (20):1449-1456, 1977.
70. Zurier RB, Gionfriddo M, Miller P: Treatment of NZB/W ("lupus") mice with 15(S)-15-methyl PGE_1. Prostaglandins Med (4):281-284, 1980.
71. Krakauer KA, Torrey SB, Zurier RB: Prostaglandin E_1 treatment of NZB/W mice. III. Preservation of spleen cell concentrations and mitogen-induced proliferative responses. Clin Immunol Immunopathol (11):256-267, 1978.
72. Winkelstein A, Kelley VE: The effects of PGE_1 on lymphocytes in NZB/W mice. Clin Immunol Immunopathol (17):212-219, 1980.
73. Kelley VE, Winkelstein A, Izui S, Dixon FJ: Prostaglandin E_1 inhibits T-cell proliferation and renal disease in MRL/l mice. Clin Immunol Immunopathol (21):190-203, 1981.
74. Chensue SW, Kunkel SL, Ward PA, Higashi G: Exogenously administered prostaglandins modulate pulmonary granulomas induced by Schistosoma mansoni eggs. Am J Pathol (111):78-81, 1983.

75. Chensue SW, Wellhausen SR, Boros DL: Modulation of granulomatous hypersensitivity. Participation of Ly1+ and Ly2+ T lymphocytes in the suppression of granuloma formation and lymphokine in the suppression of granuloma formation production in Schistosoma mansoni infected mice. J Immunol (127):363-367, 1981.
76. Chensue SW, Kunkel SL: Arachidonic acid metabolism and macrophage activation. Clin Lab Med (3):677-694, 1983.
77. DiPasquale G, Rassaert C, Righter R, Welaj P, Tripp L: Influence of PGE_2 and $PGF_{2\alpha}$ on the inflammatory process. Prostaglandins (3):741-745, 1973.
78. Bonta IL, Parnham MJ, Adolfs MJP: Reduced exudation and increased tissue proliferation during chronic inflammation in rats deprived of endogenous prostaglandin precursors. Prostaglandins (14):295-307, 1977.
79. Parnham JM, Shoshan S, Bonta IL, Neiman-Wollner S: Increased collagen metabolism in granulomata induced in rats deficient in endogenous prostaglandin precursors. Prostaglandins (14):709-714, 1977.
80. Bonta IL, Parnham JM: Time dependent stimulatory and inhibitory effects of PGE_1 on exudative and tissue components of granulomatous inflammation in rats. Br J Pharmacol (65):465-472, 1979.

Chapter 7

REGULATION OF THE IMMUNE RESPONSE BY EICOSANOID ACIDS

NORBERT GUALDE, JEAN-CLAUDE ALDIGIER, SYLVIE MEXMAIN and JAMES S. GOODWIN

1. INTRODUCTION

Oxygenated arachidonic acid derivatives are metabolites that issue from both the cyclooxygenase and the lipoxygenase pathways and act as important local immunoregulators. The cyclooxygenase products, especially the prostaglandins (PGs), are being thoroughly investigated with regard to their role in the immune response. Inhibition of lymphocyte activity is the main function of prostaglandins as immunoregulators, and PGE_2 may be viewed as a macrophage messenger for an inhibitory signal to lymphocytes (1). It is likely that PGE_2 is a biological mediator of a physiologic negative feedback mechanism following stimulation by antigens (2).

The compounds which issue from the lipoxygenase pathway, the eicosanoids, have been described more recently. In this chapter, we will review the literature linking hydroperoxyeicosatetraenoic acids (HPETEs), hydroxyeicosatetraenoic acids (HETEs) and leukotrienes (LTs) to regulation of the immune response. First, we will briefly describe the lipoxygenase cascade which leads to these eicosanoids.

2. TRANSFORMATION OF ARACHIDONIC ACID VIA THE LIPOXYGENASE PATHWAY

The term "lipoxygenase" is generally understood to denote the enzymes which catalyse the production of LTs, but the pathway which finally yields numerous LTs also gives rise to many other oxidative derivatives of arachidonic acid (3). Among the cells involved in the immune response, macrophages are more important than lymphocytes as producers of monohydroxylated fatty acids (4), and one would expect that these compounds, similarly to PGs, serve as physiological macrophage to lymphocyte messengers.

Table 1 lists the monohydroxylated fatty acids found in the supernatant after incubation of mouse peritoneal macrophages with exogenous arachidonic acid. Arachidonic acid leads to six hydroperoxyeicosatetraenoic acid precursors of monohydroxylated eicosatetraenoic acids.

Table 1. Monohydroxylated fatty acid production by mouse peritoneal macrophages.

Monohydroxylated Fatty Acids	Percentage
12 - OH - 5, 8, 10, 14 eicosatetraenoic acid	52.0
15 - OH - 5, 8, 11, 13 eicosatetraenoic acid	15.0
11 - OH - 5, 8, 12, 14 eicosatetraenoic acid	10.0
8 - OH - 5, 9, 11, 14 eicosatetraenoic acid	8.5
9 - OH - 5, 7, 11, 14 eicosatetraenoic acid	8.5
5 - OH - 6, 8, 11, 14 eicosatetraenoic acid	5.0

Leukotrienes are produced after oxidation of arachidonic acid at C-5, giving rise to an unstable compound called 5-HPETE. The steps yielding LTs via the 5-lipoxygenase pathway are summarized in Figure 1. This pathway is the most important mechanism for producing LTs, but novel alternate pathways for leukotriene formation acting with enzymes catalyzing the introduction of oxygen at C-12 and C-15 have also been described (5).

The biological activities and physiologic roles of the various lipoxygenase products are largely unknown. LTC_4, LTD_4 and LTE_4 are potent constrictors of bronchial smooth muscle, approximately four orders of magnitude more potent than histamine in this regard (5). LTC_4 and LTD_4 in doses as low as 10^{-13}M increase microvascular permeability. At slightly higher concentrations (10^{-8} to 10^{-10}M), LTC_4 and LTD_4 constrict terminal arterioles, contributing to vascular leakage (6). LTC_4, LTD_4 and LTE_4 have also been reported to contract smooth muscle of the stomach and ileum in various species and to have possible

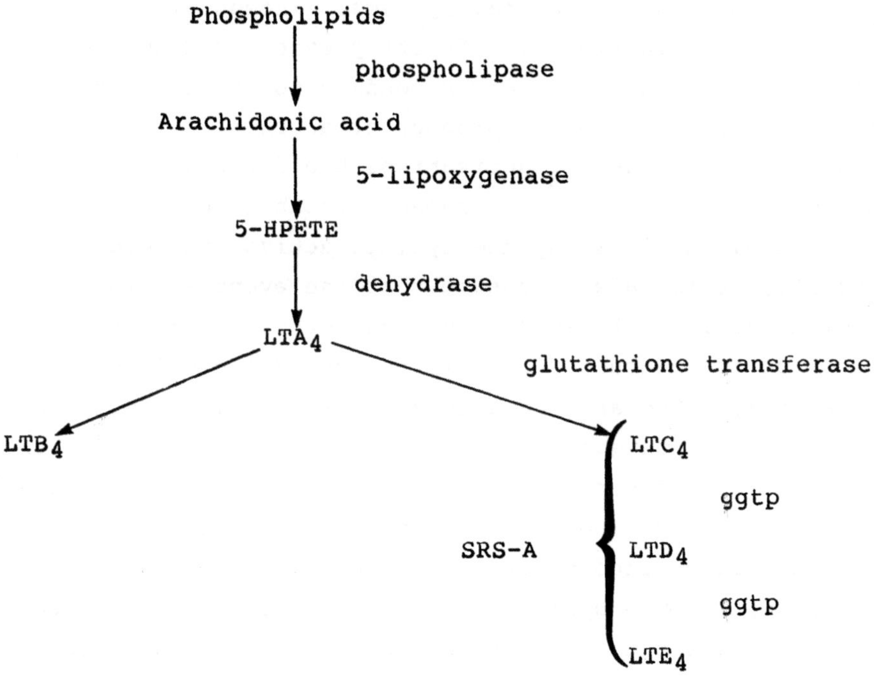

ggtp = gammaglutamyltranspeptidase
SRS-A = slow reactive substance of anaphylaxis

FIGURE 1. Metabolism of arachidonic acid via the lipoxygenase pathway.

cardiac effects (7). LTB_4 is a powerful chemoattractant and chemokinetic agent for polymorphonuclear leukocytes (PMNs) (8) and also stimulates PMN aggregation and adherence to endothelial cells (9,10). In addition, lipoxygenase inhibitors reduce, and LTB_4 stimulates, human natural killer (NK) cell activity (11). Several groups have reported that various arachidonic acid metabolites regulate the synthesis of other arachidonic acid metabolites. For example, LTC_4 stimulates leukotriene synthesis in endothelial cells (12), and 15-HETE in relatively high concentrations ($>10^{-6}$M) inhibits 5-lipoxygenase activity in some cell types (13,14) while it actually stimulates leukotriene synthesis several-fold in other cell types (15). In addition, inhibition of cyclooxygenase leads to "shunting" of arachidonic acid into the lipoxygenase pathway, resulting in increased leukotriene production in several systems. Indeed, it may well be that some of the physiologic effects previously described for cyclooxygenase inhibitors are secondary to the increased production of one lipoxygenase product or another.

Because phospholipase A_2 activation, the first step in arachidonic acid metabolism, is probably as ubiquitous a response to stimuli as is adenylate cyclase activation (e.g., Reference 16), it is safe to assume that the eventual list of biological actions of leukotrienes and other lipoxygenase metabolites of arachidonic acid will be considerably longer than it is today. One area that remains largely uninvestigated is the action of lipoxygenase metabolites in humoral and cellular immune responses. Parker and his coworkers (17-19) found that compounds which inhibit both lipoxygenases and cyclooxygenases inhibit ^{3}H-thymidine incorporation into mitogen-stimulated lymphocytes, while pure cyclooxygenase inhibitors stimulate the same response. These investigators concluded that lipoxygenase metabolites are necessary for mitogen-induced lymphocyte proliferation. Webb and associates reported that LTB_4 and LTE_4, in concentrations as low as 10^{-12}M, cause >50% inhibition of phytohemagglutinin (PHA)-induced ^{3}H-thymidine incorporation in mouse splenic T cells, while much higher concentrations (10^{-7}M) inhibit the formation of antibody-producing cells against sheep red blood cells (RBC) in Mishell-Dutton cultures (20). In contrast, in PHA-stimulated cultures of human T cells, Payan and Goetzl found no inhibition of human T cell proliferation by LTC_4 or LTD_4, but they did find some inhibition of proliferation and lymphokine production with relatively high concentrations (10^{-7}M) of LTB_4 (21). Rola-Pleszczynski et al. also reported a modest inhibition of PHA-stimulated mitogenesis in human lymphocytes by LTB_4 over a wide range of concentrations with no obvious dose response (22). More important, these authors observed that T cells preincubated with concentrations of LTB_4 as low as 10^{-12}M suppress the ^{3}H-thymidine incorporation of fresh, autologous T cells in subsequent PHA-stimuated cultures.

In 1980, it was clearly demonstrated by Goodman et al. that 15-HETE, a hydroperoxide derivative of arachidonic acid, inhibits mitogen-induced lymphocyte proliferation in vitro (23). This inhibitory effect was confirmed by Bailey et al. (13) and extended to various HPETEs (24). We examined the effects of HPETEs (24) and HETEs (25) on lectin-stimulated tritiated thymidine incorporation in mouse splenocytes (25) and in human peripheral blood mononuclear cells (PBMC) (26). We found that various HPETEs and HETEs diminish ^{3}H-thymidine uptake when added in small concentrations (10^{-6} to 10^{-10}M) to lymphocytes stimulated by concanavalin A (Con A) or PHA. When purified human T cells supplemented by 5% monocytes were stimulated by PHA or Con A in the presence of 15-HPETE which had been added at the start of the culture, a clear inhibition of proliferation was observed. As shown in Table 2, this eicosanoid-induced inhibition depended upon the lectin and/or hydroperoxide concentration (27).

Table 2. 15-HPETE inhibition of human T cell proliferation in vitro.

Mitogens	Concentration (μg/ml)	15-HPETE molar concentration 4×10^{-8}	4×10^{-7}	4×10^{-6}
		percentage of inhibition (mean ± SD)		
PHA	5	20 ± 23	43 ± 26	80 ± 18
PHA	10	6 ± 13	43 ± 34	62 ± 20
Con A	10	44 ± 30	56 ± 25	90 ± 9
Con A	20	41 ± 19	74 ± 18	94 ± 12

Therefore, it became obvious that many of the molecules produced by the lipoxygenase cascade inhibit lymphocyte proliferative response to mitogens. Suppressive activity induced in vitro by 15-HPETE and by 15-HETE was also observed during the allostimulation procedures. For instance, when C57Bl/6 responder splenocytes were cocultured with DBA/2(-)-irradiated stimulator cells, thymidine uptake by proliferating B6 clones was diminished by adding 15-HPETE or 15-HETE (24), and the subsequent generation of B6 anti-D2 killer T cells was restricted (24). The immunosuppressive activity of 15-HPETE on human T lymphocytes was studied more carefully when the cells carrying the OKT4 marker of the helper/inducer subset and the lymphocytes positive for the OKT8 marker of the suppressor/cytotoxic subset were sorted and separately stimulated with PHA or Con A in the presence of 15-HPETE (4×10^{-6} to 4×10^{-8}M). It was noticed that, in terms of proliferative response to lectins, the OKT4(+) T cells were less inhibited than the OKT8(+) T cells (28).

3. EFFECTS OF 15-HPETE ON LYMPHOCYTE MEMBRANE RECEPTORS

Human T lymphocytes carry receptors for sheep RBC and therefore bind these erythrocytes to form E rosettes (ER). We tested ER formation in 130 healthy HLA-typed blood donors after preincubation of PBMC with or without 15-HPETE (26). We observed that ER formation was inhibited when the lymphocytes had been treated with 15-HPETE for 2 h. For the 130 tested subjects, the mean value of rosette inhibition by 15-HPETE was 30 ± 15%, allowing us to separate the subjects into two groups: the first group including individuals with ER inhibition equal to or smaller than 30% (low sensitivity group) and the second including subjects with ER inhibition higher than 30% (high sensitivity group). In these two populations, we observed a difference according to the HLA-A29 and B12 phenotypes (the genes corresponding to these antigens are often associated on the sixth chromosome by a linkage disequilibrium). The non-B12 subjects were equally distributed between the two groups (Table 3), but most of the B12(+) subjects belonged to the low sensitivity group and were simultaneously A29(-). These results suggest that, with respect to 15-HPETE sensitivity, either A29 and B12 are epistatic genes, or the sixth chromosome possesses a gene (absent from the B12[+] A29[-] haplotype) which increases sensitivity to 15-HPETE.

It is likely that 15-HPETE induces a loss of sheep RBC receptors by human T lymphocytes. We also observed that incubation of human T lymphocytes with 15-HPETE resulted in diminution of 1) the number of receptors for the Fc fragment of IgG on the so-called Tγ cells and 2) the number of T lymphocytes carrying this type of receptor (29). These modifications affecting two types of T cell receptors might be caused by the changes in lymphocyte membrane fluidity induced by both 15-HPETE and 15-HETE.

Table 3. 15-HPETE inhibition of sheep rosette formation by human lymphocytes.*

Group of subjects§	Percentage of subjects with respect to the HLA-A29 and B12 phenotypes			
	A29- B12-	A29+ B12-	A29+ B12+	A29- B12+
1	31	4	5	17#
2	30	4	7	2

*Distribution of 130 subjects according to their sensitivity to 15-HPETE and their HLA-A29 and B12 phenotype.

§Group 1 = low sensitivity, group 2 = high sensitivity to 15-HPETE.

#$\chi^2 = 12.33$, $p = 0.006$.

4. MODIFICATIONS OF LYMPHOCYTE MEMBRANE FLUIDITY BY MONOHYDROXYLATED FATTY ACIDS

We measured the viscosity of the lymphocyte membrane using a polarization fluorescence technique (30). A fluorescent probe, 1,6 diphenyl-1,3,5-hexatriene, was embedded in the phospholipid core of the lymphocyte membrane, and the motion of this probe was analyzed by fluorescence polarization. The in vitro effect of 15-HETE (4×10^{-8} to 2×10^{-7}M) was very fast and resulted in a tremendous increase of viscosity, from 1.62 to 2.75 poise units, and a dramatic increase in the degree of order, from 0.49 to 0.79, one being the theoretical maximum for degree of order.

5. INDUCTION OF SUPPRESSOR CELLS BY 15-HPETE AND 15-HETE

We preincubated B6 lymphocytes for 24 h in culture media with or without 15-HPETE or 15-HETE. When added to cocultures of fresh B6 cells and D2-irradiated stimulator cells, the treated cells partially inhibited the proliferative response of the B6 cells (31). One possible explanation for this result is that mouse lymphocytes incubated with 15-HPETE or 15-HETE acquire a suppressive activity.

The same phenomenon was observed with human T cells (32). Purified human T cells preincubated with 15-HPETE no longer supported immunoglobulin production by fresh, autologous, pokeweed mitogen (PWM)-stimulated B cells in the presence of fresh, autologous T lymphocytes.

We extended these observations on the phenotypic nature of eicosanoid-induced mouse and human suppressor cells. When mouse splenocytes were incubated in vitro for 48 h with 15-HETE (10^{-5} to 10^{-8}M final concentration), we noticed an increase in the percentage of cells carrying the Lyt-2(+) antigen (33) (Table 4).

Table 4. Modification of splenocyte Lyt markers by 15-HETE.

Preincubation	Lyt-1(+)2(-) cells	Lyt-1(-)2(+) cells
media	30 ± 8	8 ± 3
15-HETE	35 ± 6	14 ± 5

We also observed that when human T cells were similarly preincubated with 15-HPETE and were treated with an anti-OKT8 monoclonal antibody plus complement, the suppression of IgG production was eliminated. However, when the suppressor OKT8(+) cells were eliminated before the preincubation, the generation of new suppressor cells by 15-HPETE was not affected (32).

A possible explanation for the above data is that 15-HPETE and 15-HETE might convert a population of non-suppressor lymphocytes to a subset of suppressor cells. For instance, 15-HPETE might change OKT8(-) presuppressor T cells into OKT8(+) suppressor cells. This hypothesis is sustained by the following experiment.

T cells and OKT8(-) T cells were incubated separately for 24 h with or without 15-HPETE. The percentage of cells bearing suppressor surface markers was then determined by flow microfluorograph analysis following incubation with a directly fluoresceinated antibody. In the OKT8(-) T cell populations treated by 15-HPETE, we observed a large increase in suppressor OKT8(+) cells (32).

The problem was then to determine if the increase in the percentage of cells carrying suppressor surface markers was merely a membrane phenomenon resulting from the expression or relocation of hidden OKT8 or Lyt-2 antigens or if it was a mechanism related to cell proliferation and differentiation. We therefore studied the cell cycle of 15-HETE-treated lymphocytes using flow microfluorograph analysis of nuclear DNA following ethidium bromide staining. We observed that 15-HETE increased the percentage of cells in the G_2 phase after 41 h of preincubation and that this increment was preceded from the 17th to the 22nd hour by an increase of cells in the S phase.

6. IMMUNOSUPPRESSION INDUCED IN VIVO BY 15-HETE

C57Bl/6 mice were injected daily intraperitoneally with 250 µg of 15-HETE for 7 d. This treatment diminished 1) thymidine uptake by PHA-stimulated and Con A-stimulated splenocytes and 2) proliferation induced by mixed lymphocyte reaction. It was also observed that lymphocytes from the B6-treated mice diminished the alloreactivity of B6 cells from the control animals (33).

7. ENHANCEMENT OF THE IMMUNE RESPONSE BY EICOSANOIDS IN VITRO

Increased NK activity in vitro in the presence of LTB_4 is, so far, the only case described of enhanced immune response induced by a product of lipoxygenation (11). Since PGs inhibit this natural cytotoxicity, Rola-Pleszczynsky et al. speculate that NK activity is regulated by a balance between products issued from the cyclooxygenase and lipoxygenase pathways (34).

8. MECHANISM(S) OF EICOSANOID-INDUCED IMMUNOSUPPRESSION

There is a good deal of evidence that lipoxygenase arachidonic acid metabolites suppress the immune response, but the mechanism of this immunosuppression is not yet clear.

It is possible that these lipoxigenic metabolites can affect an entire lymphocyte population merely by altering the physical properties of the lymphocytes. We observed that both 15-HPETE and 15-HETE dramatically modify the viscosity of the plasmatic membranes of splenocytes, as mentioned above (27). Thus, there is a chance that 15-HPETE and 15-HETE suppress in vitro lymphocyte activity by causing rigidity of the lymphocyte membranes, thereby blocking receptor mobility, which is necessary for the initiation of mitogenesis.

It was also observed by Bailey et al. (13) that 15-HETE modifies lymphocyte metabolism somewhat, mostly inhibiting 12-HETE synthesis. In addition, it is well known that 15-HPETE inhibits the synthesis of PGI_2 (35), and Honn et al. postulated that the increase in tumor metastasis observed after intravenous injection of 15-HPETE is caused by enhanced platelet aggregation resulting from the decrease in PGI_2 synthesis (36).

Hydroperoxy acids cause a rise in the level of intracellular cyclic guanylate monophosphate (cGMP) (37), a phenomenon usually associated with enhanced cell activities, such as lymphocyte proliferation (38). According to our preliminary data, 15-HETE increases lymphocyte cGMP (39). If this is true, the effects of 15-HETE on lymphocyte metabolism are quite contradictory, i.e., 1) augmentation of cGMP, which gives rise to proliferation, and 2) inhibition of 12-HETE production, which leads to immunosuppression (13). However, changes in the physical state of the cell membrane or in cell metabolism cannot explain how the sensitivity of human lymphocytes to 15-HPETE is HLA-linked (26) or why OKT8(+) cells are less sensitive to 15-HPETE than the

OKT4(+) cell subset with regard to mitogen-induced thymidine uptake (26).

Rola-Pleszczynsky et al. observed that the immunosuppression induced by LTB_4 is related to the generation of immunosuppressive cells (22), and it is likewise probable that eicosanoid-induced immunosuppression involves more than cell metabolism or the physical state of the cell membranes. Since we observed contradictory phenomena induced by 15-HPETE and by 15-HETE, namely, inhibition of the proliferative response of lymphocytes versus augmentation of intracellular cGMP and the synthesis of DNA, we speculate that both 15-HPETE and 15-HETE induce differentiation and proliferation of a subset of pre-suppressor cells, giving rise to suppressor OKT8(+) or Lyt-2(+) lymphocytes. If this hypothesis is correct, the increase in the level of cGMP and in the synthesis of DNA is related to the proliferation of the suppressor subset.

9. CONCLUSION

The eicosanoids involved in regulating the immune response are produced mostly by macrophages. Since their half life is very brief, it is likely that these metabolites act as local immunoregulators remaining in the environment of the producer cells. The majority of molecules studied with respect to their effects on lymphocytes are immunosuppressive essentially, but not exclusively, by inducing suppressor cells.

REFERENCES

1. Goodwin JS, Webb DR: Regulation of the immune response by prostaglandins. Clin Immunol Immunopathol (15): 106-122, 1980.
2. Goodwin JS, Ceuppens JL, Gualde N: Control of the immune response in humans by prostaglandins. In: Otterness I, Capetola RJ, Wong S (eds) Therapeutic control of inflammatory diseases. Raven Press, New York, 1983, pp 79 to 92.
3. Rabinovitch H, Durand J, Gualde N, Rigaud M: Metabolism of polyunsaturated fatty acids by mouse peritoneal macrophages: the lipoxygenase metabolic pathway. Agents Actions (11): 580-583, 1981.

4. Rigaud M, Durand J, Breton JC: Transformation of arachidonic acid into 12-hydroxy-5,8,10,14-eicosatetraenoic acid by mouse peritoneal macrophages. Biochim Biophys Acta (573): 408-412, 1979.
5. Samuelsson B: Leukotrienes: mediators of immediate hypersensitivity reactions and inflammation. Science (220): 568-575, 1983.
6. Dahlén SE, Björk J, Hedqvist P, Arfors KE, Hammarström S, Lindgren JA, Samuelsson B: Leukotrienes promote plasma leakage and leukocyte adhesion in postcapillary venules: in vivo effects with relevance to the acute inflammatory response. Proc Natl Acad Sci USA (78): 3887-3891, 1981.
7. Hammarström S: Leukotrienes. Annu Rev Biochem (52): 355-377, 1983.
8. Ford-Hutchinson AW, Bray MA, Doig MV, Shipley ME, Smith MJH: Leukotriene B, a potent chemokinetic and aggregating substance released from polymorphonuclear leukocytes. Nature (286): 264-265, 1980.
9. Goetzl EJ, Brindley LL, Goldman DW: Enhancement of human neutrophil adherence by synthetic leukotriene constituents of the slow-reacting substance of anaphylaxis. Immunology (50): 35-42, 1983.
10. Lewis RA, Austen KF: Mediation of local homeostasis and inflammation by leukotrienes and other mast cell-dependent compounds. Nature (293): 103-108, 1981.
11. Rola-Pleszczynski M, Gagnon L, Sirois P: Leukotriene B_4 augments human natural cytotoxic cell activity. Biochem Biophys Res Commun (113): 531-537, 1983.
12. Benjamin CW, Hopkins NK, Oglesby T, Gorman R: Against specific desensitization of leukotriene C_4-stimulated PGI_2 synthesis in human endothelial cells. Biochem Biophys Res Commun (117): 780-787, 1983.
13. Bailey JM, Bryant RW, Low CE, Pupillo MB, Vanderhoek JY: Regulation of T lymphocyte mitogenesis by the leukocyte product 15-hydroxyeicosatetraenoic acid (15-HETE). Cell Immunol (67): 112-120, 1982.
14. Vanderhoek JY, Bryant RW, Bailey JM: Inhibition of leukotriene biosynthesis by the leukocyte product 15-hydroxyeicosatetraenoic acid. J Biol Chem (255): 10064-10065, 1980.
15. Vanderhoek JY, Tare NS, Bailey M, Goldstein A, Pluznik D: New role for 15-hydroxyeicosatetraenoic acid. J Biol Chem (257): 12191-12195, 1982.
16. Crews FT, Morita Y, McGivney A, Hirata F, Siraganian RP, Axelrod J: IgE-mediated histamine release in rat basophilic leukemia cells: receptor activation, phospholipid methylation, Ca^2 flux, and release of arachidonic acid. Arch Biochem Biophys (212): 561-571, 1981.
17. Kelly JP, Parker CW: Effects of arachidonic acid and other unsaturated fatty acids on mitogenesis in human lymphocytes. J Immunol (122): 1556-1562, 1979.

18. Kelly JP, Johnson MC, Parker CW: Effect of inhibitors of arachidonic acid metabolism on mitogenesis in human lymphocytes: possible role of thromboxanes and products of the lipoxygenase pathway. J Immunol (122): 1563-1571, 1979.
19. Parker CW, Stenson WF, Huber MG, Kelly JP: Formation of thromboxane B_2 and hydroxyarachidonic acids in purified human lymphocytes in the presence and absence of PHA. J Immunol (122): 1572-1577, 1979.
20. Webb DR, Nowowiejski I, Healy C, Rogers TJ: Immunosuppressive properties of leukotriene D_4 and E_4 in vitro. Biochem Biophys Res Commun (104): 1617-1622, 1982.
21. Payan DG, Goetzl EJ: Specific suppression of human T lymphocyte function by leukotriene B_4. J Immunol (131): 551-553, 1983.
22. Rola-Pleszczynski M, Borgeat P, Sirois P: Leukotriene B_4 induces human suppressor lymphocytes. Biochem Biophys Res Commun (108): 1531-1537, 1982.
23. Goodman MG, Weigle WO: Inhibition of lymphocyte mitogenesis by an arachidonic acid hydroperoxide. J Supramol Struct (13): 373-383, 1980.
24. Gualde N, Rigaud M, Rabinovitch H, Durand J, Beneytout JL, Breton JC: Inhibition de la résponse lymphocytaire par les métabolites libérés par la lipoxygénase des macrophages chez la souris. C R Seances Acad Sci [III] (Paris) (293): 359-362 (Eng. Abstr.), 1981.
25. Gualde N, Chable-Rabinovitch H, Motta C, Durand J, Beneytout JL, Rigaud M: Hydroperoxyeicosatetraenoic acids--potent inhibitors of lymphocyte responses. Biochim Biophys Acta (750): 429-433, 1983.
26. Gualde N, Rabinovitch H, Fredon M, Rigaud M: Effects of 15-hydroperoxyeicosatetraenoic acid on human lymphocyte sheep erythrocyte rosette formation and response to Concanavalin A associated with HLA system. Eur J Immunol (12): 773-777, 1982.
27. Gualde N: Les métabolites oxygénés de l'acide arachidonique et l'activité des lymphocytes. PhD thesis in immunology, Université Paris VI, Paris, 1983.
28. Gualde N, Goodwin JS, Chable-Rabinovitch H, Beneytout JL, Shinitzki M, Rigaud M: Fifth international congress of immunology, Kyoto, 1983.
29. Goodwin JS, Gualde N, Aldigier J, Rigaud M, Vanderhoek JY: Modulation of Fcγ receptors on T cells and monocytes by 15 hydroperoxyeicosatetraenoic acid. Prostaglandins Med (13): 109-112, 1984.
30. Gualde N: First international workshop on lipoxygenase and animal tissues, Limoges, 1983.
31. Aldigier JC, Gualde N, Mexmain S, Chable-Rabinovitch H, Ratinaud MH, Rigaud M: Immunosuppression induced in vivo by 15 hydroxyeicosatetraenoic acid (15 HETE). Prostaglandins Med (13): 99-107, 1984.
32. Gualde N, Rigaud M, Goodwin JS: Induction of suppressor cells from human peripheral blood T cells by 15 hydroperoxyeicosatetraenoic acid (15 HPETE). Clin Res (31): 490A, 1983.

33. Mexmain S, Gualde N, Aldigier JC, Motta C, Chable-Rabinovitch H, Rigaud M: Specific binding of 15 HETE to lymphocytes. Effects on the fluidity of plasmatic membranes. Prostaglandins Med (13): 93-97, 1984.
34. Rola-Pleszczynski M, Gagnon L, Sirois P: International meeting on eicosanoids and cancer, Bandor, 1983.
35. Salmon JA, Smith DR, Flower RJ, Moncada S, Vane JR: Further studies on the enzymatic conversion of prostaglandin endoperoxide into prostacyclin by porcine aorta microsomes. Biochim Biophys Acta (523): 250-262, 1978.
36. Honn KV, Busse WD, Sloane BF: Prostacyclin and thromboxanes --implications for their role in tumor cell metastasis. Biochem Pharmacol (32): 1-11, 1983.
37. Harbon S, Leiber D, Vesin M-F: Phospholipase A_2 activation coupled to lipoxygenase and cyclooxygenase pathways in the guinea pig myometrium: interaction with the cyclic AMP and cyclic GMP systems. In: Samuelsson B, Paoletti R, Ramwell PW (eds) Advances in prostaglandin, thromboxane, and leukotriene research, Vol. 12. Raven Press, New York, 1983, pp 423-428.
38. Strom TB, Lundin AP, Carpenter CB: The role of cyclic nucleotides in lymphocyte activation and function. In: Schwartz RS (ed) Progress in clinical immunology, Vol. 3. Grune and Stratton, New York, 1977, pp 115-153.
39. Gualde N, Mexmain S, Aldigier JC, Goodwin JS, Rigaud M: Eicosanoids and the immune response. In: Craste de Paulet J (ed) Eicosanoids and cancer. Raven Press, New York, in press.

Chapter 8

REGULATION OF PROSTAGLANDIN SYNTHESIS BY BIOLOGICAL RESPONSE MODIFIERS AND EFFECT ON NATURAL KILLER CELLS AND BONE MARROW

MICHAEL A. CHIRIGOS, ERICH SCHLICK AND KLAUS HARTUNG

1. INTRODUCTION

Prostaglandins of the E-series (PGE) have been shown to have numerous effects on the cellular components of the immune system (for review see 1). PGE modulates the cytotoxicity of natural killer (NK) cells (2, 3) and also has been suggested to serve as a negative feedback regulator of macrophage-mediated cytotoxicity (4, 5). Immunoglobulin production by B cells is augmented by PGE (6), whereas blastogenesis of T cells after mitogen stimulation and cell-mediated immunity are inhibited by PGE (7, 8, 9). Growth and differentiation of the granulocyte-macrophage-committed stem cell (GM-CFU-C) in the bone marrow appears to be regulated by the antagonistic effects of colony-stimulating factor and PGE (10). Additionally, PGE production by tumor cells has been suggested to be a mechanism by which tumor cells can escape the host's immune surveillance (11). The major source for PGE in the immune system has been shown to be monocytes and macrophages (Mϕ) (12). When stimulated with different agents, such as lipopolysaccharide (LPS) and zymosan, mononuclear phagocytes increase their PGE production and release high amounts of PGE (5, 13, 14). Several biological response modifiers (BRMs) have been reported to be Mϕ activators and some also augment NK cells (for review see 15). A few have also been shown to activate naive macrophages directly in vitro to express a tumoricidal response. Few studies have been conducted to assess whether BRMs, reported to be Mϕ activators, could alter PGE production.

J.S. Goodwin (ed.), PROSTAGLANDINS AND IMMUNITY.

In view of the recent interest in the use of BRMs in cancer treatment, either as a monotherapy or in conjunction with cytoreductive therapy, it was of interest to test a few agents of potential usefulness in cancer therapy for their effect on PGE production by murine and human macrophages and bone marrow and the effect of PGE on the growth of GM-CFU-C stem cells and NK cell activity.

2. MATERIALS AND METHODS

2.1. Murine macrophages (mMϕ)

Peritoneal mMϕ were aseptically harvested from male BALB/c mice, 8 to 10 wk old, supplied by the Mammalian Genetics and Animal Production Section, DCT, NCI, NIH, Frederick, MD. Three x 10^5 resident peritoneal mMϕ were seeded onto 16-mm wells (Costar, Cambridge, MA) in 1 ml of RPMI 1640 medium (GIBCO, Grand Island, NY) supplemented with 10% heat-inactivated fetal calf serum (GIBCO), 125 μg/ml gentamycin (Sigma Chemical Co., St. Louis, MO) and 292 μg/ml L-glutamine (GIBCO) (RPMI-FCS). The cultures were incubated for 2 h and the adherent mMϕ-monolayers (> 95% Mϕ as determined by esterase and Wright's staining) were washed twice with medium before use in experiments.

2.2. Human blood monocytes (hM)

Human monocytes were obtained by elutriation from leukapheresis cell suspension as previously described (16). The purity of the hM was 93% (16). The hM were suspended at a concentration of 10^6 cells/ml in RPMI 1640 medium containing 10% heat-inactivated pooled human AB serum (RPMI-ABS).

2.3. BRMs

Polyriboinosinic-polycytidylic acid complexed with poly-L-lysine and stabilized with carboxymethyl cellulose (poly ICLC) was kindly supplied by Dr. H.B. Levy (NIAID, NIH, Frederick, MD). Maleic anhydride divinyl ether copolymer (MVE-2) was kindly supplied by Dr. R. Corrano (Adria Laboratories, Columbus, OH). The 2-cyanoaziridines, Azimexon

(2-[2-cyanoaziridinyl-(1)]-2-[2-carbamoylaziridinyl-(1)] propane) and BM 41.332 (2-cyano-1-[cyano-1-[2-methoxy-6-methyl-pyridine-3yl)-methyl]-aziridine, were generously provided by Dr. U. Bicker (Boehringer GmbH, Mannheim, Germany). Lipopolysaccharide from Salmonella typhimurium (LPS) was purchased from DIFCO (Detroit, MI). Murine interferon (mIFN) used: mαβIFN (Bionetics Laboratory Products, Kensington, MD).

2.3.1. Human IFNs. Partially purified preparations of natural leukocyte ($hIFN_{\alpha}$ Leuk; specific activity: 4×10^6 U/mg protein) were obtained from the Antiviral Substances Program, NIAID, NIH, Bethesda, MD. Partially purified fibroblast IFN ($hIFN_{\beta}$; specific activity: 7×10^6 U/mg protein) was purchased from HEM Research (Rockville, MD). Purified recombinant $hIFN_{\gamma}$ from Escherichia coli (specific activity: 1.7×10^7 U/mg protein) was a generous gift from Dr. P. Gray, Genentech (San Francisco, CA). BM 41.332 was initially dissolved in absolute ethanol and further diluted with complete medium. The final ethanol concentrations were $< 0.1\%$ and had no influence on PGE production (data not shown). All other drugs were directly dissolved in complete medium.

2.4. Murine bone marrow cells (mBMC)

Sterile single-cell suspensions from femoral bone marrow were prepared as previously described (17). Bone marrow mononuclear cells were separated by centrifugation on Ficoll-Hypaque. Adherent mononuclear bone marrow cells were removed by plastic adherence. Morphological characterization of the bone marrow cells was done by Giemsa and esterase staining. 10^7 mononuclear bone marrow cells were then incubated in 1 ml complete medium in 16-mm wells (Costar).

2.5. PGE-radioimmunoassay

PGE was determined by radioimmunoassay as previously described (18, 19). PGE_2 was purchased from Upjohn Corp. (Kalamazoo, MI) and initially dissolved in absolute ethanol. Further dilutions were made in Tris-buffer (0.83% NaCl and 0.12% Trizma pH 7.4). ^3H-PGE_2 (Tracer, spec. activity: 165

Ci/mmol) was obtained from New England Nuclear (Boston, MA). Antibody to PGE_2 was purchased from Accurate Chemicals (Westbury, NY). The cross-reactivity of the antibody was: PGE_2 100%, PGE_1 60%, PGA_2 10%, PGB_2 1.5%, $PGF_{1\alpha}$ 2%, 13,14 dihydro-15 keto PGE_2 1%. Because of the high cross-reactivity of the antibody with PGE_1, all values are expressed as PGE. Antibody and tracer were diluted in Tris-buffer with 0.1% gelatin (#G7, Fisher, NJ). 0.05% dextran (Pharmacia, Uppsala)-coated charcoal (0.5%, Norit A, Fisher) was used to separate the ligand from free PGE. 100 µl of sample was incubated at room temperature with 50 µl of antibody for 2 h. 50 µl of tracer (~ 9,000 cpm) was added, vortexed and incubated at 4°C for 16 h. Then 250 µl of 1% gelatin and 500 µl of iced charccal-dextran were added and vortexed, and the vials were allowed to sit at 4°C for 20 min. After centrifugation at 500 g for 10 min, supernatants were decanted into scintillation vials, 15 ml of Insta-gel (Packard, Warrinville, IL) were added, and samples were counted in a β-scintillation counter (Nuclear, Chicago, IL). Double determinations were always performed, and samples with PGE concentrations exceeding the linear part of the standard curve were reassayed after further dilution with medium. The medium did not have any nonspecific binding properties. The detection limit of the RIA was 10 pg PGE/0.1 ml sample.

To make values comparable, all the results are expressed as ng PGE produced by 10^5 cells. This is based upon a linear relationship between the number of hM or mMϕ (10^5 to 2×10^6 cells) plated and the amount of PGE being produced (12 and our unpublished data). Student's *t*-test was used for statistical analysis.

2.6. Colony stimulating factor (CSF) assay

CSF content in cell-free conditioned medium from Mϕ/monocyte and bone marrow cells was determined as previously described (20, 21). Briefly, 10^5 nonadherent bone marrow cells were suspended in 2 ml of 0.3% agar; supplemented with 15% horse serum (GIBCO, Grand Island, NY), 15% fetal calf serum (GIBCO), and 125 μg/ml gentamycin (Sigma); and plated in 35-mm petri dishes (Falcon, Oxnard, CA). As CSF source, 0.2 ml supernatant from WEHI-3 cells (21) was used. The cultures were incubated at 37°C in a fully humidifed atmosphere of 7% CO_2 in air. Colonies (> 40 cells) were scored and classified on the basis of their morphology at day 10 of the culture period.

2.7. Natural killer (NK) cell assay

The NK cell assay was conducted as previously described (22). Briefly, various concentrations of spleen cells were incubated with 1×10^4 ^{51}Cr-labeled target cells (200 μCi/10^6 cells, 37°C water bath, 1 h) for 4 h at 37°C in round-bottomed 96-well plastic microtiter plates. After incubation the supernatant was removed by the Titertek automatic harvesting system and counted in a γ-scintillation counter. All combinations were performed in triplicate. YAC-1, a tissue culture cell line of YAC, a Moloney virus-induced lymphoma of A/Su origin, was used as the target for NK activity. The percent cytotoxicity was calculated from the formula:

$$\% \text{ cytotoxicity} = \frac{\text{experiment CPM} - \text{SR CPM}}{\text{MR CPM} - \text{SR CPM}} \times 100$$

SR = spontaneous release as determined by incubation of 1×10^4 ^{51}Cr-labeled target cells without effector cells.
MR = maximum release as determined by incubation of 1×10^4 ^{51}Cr-labeled target cells with 0.5% SDS suspension.

3. RESULTS

Table 1 shows the PGE levels in the culture fluids after 1 to 4 days of incubation of mMϕ with the optimal concentration of each BRM. Peak levels of PGE were found after 24 h. This observation suggested that either PGE production by mMϕ occurred only during the first 24 h of culture or that feedback inhibition or degradation of PGE prevented the levels from continuing to rise. To determine whether the mMϕ retained the ability to produce PGE for a longer period, we incubated mMϕ for 24 h with BRMs and subsequently washed them three times with PBS. Then either fresh RPMI-FCS or RPMI-FCS containing the BRM concentrations which were previously used was added, to determine whether there would be further production or additional stimulation of PGE release by re-exposure to these BRMs. Results indicate that the amounts of PGE released during the additional 24-h incubation period (i.e., between 24-48 h) were markedly lower than those released during the first incubation period (0-24 h) (data not shown).

Table 1. PGE secretion by peritoneal murine Mϕ after incubation with BRMs.*

BRM	Concentration per ml	Day of assay† 1	2	3	4
Medium		4.9	4.0	3.7	4.5
LPS	1 μg	12.0§	10.8§	10.4§	12.2§
Poly ICLC	1 μg	8.5§	8.0§	7.2§	8.3§
mαβIFN	100 U	8.9§	6.8§	7.5§	7.0§
Azimexon	50 μg	6.4‡	5.3	6.7‡	6.5
BM41.332	25 μg	8.0§	7.1§	6.7‡	5.8
MVE-2	50	5.2	4.4	5.0	3.9

*Three x 10^5 mMϕ were incubated in 2 ml RPMI-FCS for 1,2,3 or 4 days. Supernatants were assayed for PGE at each time period.
†ng PGE/10^5 cells
Results significantly different from medium control mMϕ: ‡$p < 0.01$; §$p < 0.001$.

Murine bone marrow cells (mBMC) were incubated with various concentrations of four BRMs. The optimal concentrations eliciting the most significant levels of PGE (Table 2) were higher than the concentrations found to be optimal for murine Mϕs. In addition, the peak levels of PGE were found after 48 h incubation. In each case, there was a significant elevation of PGE secretion, particularly for poly ICLC, mαβIFN and LPS.

Table 2. PGE secretion by murine bone marrow cells after incubation with BRMs.*

BRM	Concentration per ml	PGE ng/10^6 BMC
Medium	-	0.20
Poly ICLC	50 µg	0.55†
MVE-2	25 µg	0.28†
mαβIFN	500 U	0.60†
LPS	5 µg	0.90†

*One x 10^7 unfractionated bone marrow cells were incubated in 1 ml of RPMI-FCS with the individual BRM for 48 h and PGE concentrations in the supernatants were determined.
†Results significantly different from medium control murine bone marrow cells, $P = < 0.01$.

Since some BRMs, and particularly poly ICLC and LPS, stimulate secretion of PGE by murine Mφs and bone marrow cells (Table 1 and 2), we investigated whether this would also occur with human peripheral blood monocytes and bone marrow cells. Human monocytes spontaneously secreted about 6 ng PGE/10^6 cells when kept in complete medium for 2 days (Table 3). LPS and poly ICLC caused a significant increase in PGE secretion by both monocytes and bone marrow cells. None of the hIFNs at the concentrations tested had any influence on PGE secretion by either of the two cell populations. Since there was a concomitant increase in PGE after treatment with LPS and poly ICLC, monocytes and bone marrow cells were incubated with or without indomethacin (10^{-7} molar) for 3 h to inhibit the cyclooxygenase pathway. Poly ICLC (50 µg/ml) was then added to the cultures, and after an additional 40 h incubation, their supernatants were tested for PGE. Indomethacin completely blocked secretion of PGE by control and BRM-treated monocytes and bone marrow cells (data not shown).

Murine resident peritoneal macrophages spontaneously secrete about 4-5 ng PGE/10^5 cells when incubated in vitro. Since there was a significant increase in PGE production by murine Mφs after in vitro incubation with BRMs (Table 1),

Table 3. Secretion of PGE by human peripheral blood monocytes and bone marrow cells.

		PGE($ng/10^6$ cells)	
BRM	Concentration per ml	Bone marrow cell*	Blood monocytes*
Medium		0.31 ± 0.07	5.8 ± 0.5
Poly ICLC	50 μg	0.99 ± 0.1†	10.1 ± 0.9†
Leuk hIFNα	1 U	0.28 ± 0.06	5.2 ± 0.6
hIFNβ	10 U	0.39 ± 0.09	6.2 ± 0.4
hIFNγ	1 U	0.34 ± 0.08	6.1 ± 0.6
LPS	5 μg	1.4 ± 0.2†	8.9 ± 1.2†

*One x 10^7 Ficoll-Hypaque separated human bone marrow cells or 1 x 10^6 elutriated human peripheral blood monocytes were incubated in 1 ml of complete medium for 48 h in the presence of the indicated BRM.
†Significantly different from medium controls $P = <0.001$.

it was of interest to test the effect of the indomethacin inhibitor of the PGE biosynthetic pathway to assess its effect on the release of two Mϕ secretory products. Murine Mϕs were therefore incubated with or without indomethacin at a concentration of 10^{-7} M for 3 h to inhibit the cyclooxygenase pathway. The BRMs were then added to the Mϕ cultures and after an additional 48 h incubation, their supernatants were tested for the presence of granulocyte macrophage-colony stimulating factor (GM-CSF) and PGE. The results in Table 4 indicate that indomethacin blocked the secretion of PGE by control Mϕ as well as by Mϕ incubated concomitantly with BRMs. Indomethacin, however, did not alter the capacity of BRMs to induce GM-CSF secretion and had no significant stimulatory influence of its own on the release of GM-CSF by Mϕ.

Murine bone marrow cells were also incubated directly with different concentrations of PGE_2 (10^{-6} to 10^{-10} M) to determine its inhibitory potential for bone marrow colony growth. Results in Table 5 indicate that PGE_2 only at

Table 4. Effect of indomethacin on BRM-induced secretion of GM-CSF and PGE by murine Mϕ.*

BRM	GM-CSF (U/ml) BRM	GM-CSF (U/ml) Indo. 10^{-7} M	PGE (ng/10^5 Mϕ) BRM	PGE (ng/10^5 Mϕ) Indo. 10^{-7} M
Medium	30	32	5	1.0
mαβIFN 500 U/ml	112†	132†	8†	1.3
LPS 10 μg/ml	135†	141†	9.5†	3.0‡
Poly ICLC 50 μg/ml	124†	145†	8.3†	1.2
BM 41.332 25 μg/ml	58‡	70‡	6.5‡	1.1
MVE-2 25 μg/ml	20	28	5.5	1.0

*Resident peritoneal Mϕ (8 x 10^5) were incubated with/without indomethacin (Indo.) at 10^{-7} M for 3 h. They were then additionally incubated with either one of the BRMs for 48 h. Their supernatants were harvested and tested for GM-CSF and PGE.

†$P < 0.001$

‡$P < 0.02$ compared to medium control

concentrations greater than 10^{-8} M significantly inhibited the CSF-supported growth of granulocyte-macrophage committed bone marrow stem cell (GM-CFV-C).

Several chemical and biological agents (biological response modifiers [BRM]) have been reported to stimulate NK cell tumor cytotoxicity (23, 24). For optimal therapeutic efficacy, sustained or repeated augmentation of effector cell function is desirable. A recent phase I clinical study (25) and preclinical study (26) indicate that multiple treatment with interferon (IFN) failed to boost NK activity. In addition, we have previously reported that multiple injections of mice with maleic anhydride divinyl ether (MVE-2) induced hyporesponsiveness of spleen NK cells (27) in contrast to the significant augmentation of NK activity attained with a single injection (27, 28).

In this study, we examined the effect of indomethacin in mice receiving single or multiple treatments with MVE-2 to assess what effect the cyclooxygenase inhibitor would have on

Table 5. Inhibitory effect of PGE_2 on GM-CFU-C growth in soft agar culture.

PGE_2 concentration per culture dish	Colonies/10^5 plated bone marrow cells*	
	WEHI-3 CSF†	Mϕ-derived CSF‡
Medium	36 ± 3.5	30 ± 2.1
10^{-10} M	35 ± 4.1 (-3)	31 ± 2.7 (+3)
10^{-9} M	35 ± 2.8 (-3)	30 ± 3.3 (+0)
10^{-8} M	33 ± 2.9 (-8)	28 ± 2.3 (-7)
10^{-7} M	28 ± 2.2 (-22)§	25 ± 2.4 (-17)§
10^{-6} M	24 ± 2.4 (-33)§	21 ± 2.1 (-30)§

*10^5 nonadherent bone marrow cells were plated in 2 ml of 0.3% agar (15% FCS + 15% HS) for 10 d. Mean values ± SE of two separate experiments with four cultures each. Numbers in parentheses indicate % change compared to the medium control.

†50 μl of the appropriate concentration of PGE_2 continued in medium and 150 μl of WEHI-3 CSF (dialyzed supernatant from WEHI-3 cells with no detectable PGE levels) were added to the agar before plating.

‡ 8 x 10^5 resident peritoneal Mϕ were incubated for 2 d with 10 μg/ml LPS. The supernatant was dialyzed, ultrafiltered and concentrated using a Diaflo Ultrafilter UM10. 150 μl of this Mϕ derived and filtered supernatant (no detectable PGE) was added together with 50 μl of the appropriate concentration of PGE_2 contained in medium to the agar before plating.

§$P < 0.002$ as compared to the medium control.

the hyporesponsiveness of NK cells induced by multiple treatments with MVE-2 (Table 6). Single treatment resulted in a significant increase in NK cell cytotoxicity (grp. 2); however, multiple treatments resulted in a hyporesponsiveness to further NK cell augmentation (grp. 4). In contrast, when indomethacin was administered concomitantly with single or multiple treatments with MVE-2, a more highly elevated augmentation was attained. Of particular interest was the further augmentation occurring in mice receiving one treatment with MVE-2 (grp. 3). Indomethacin alone did not affect NK cell activity.

Table 6. Influence of indomethacin on natural killer cell response to single versus multiple treatment with MVE-2.

Group no.	Treatment Schedule* MVE-2	Indomethacin	Cytotoxicity %†
1	-	-	10
2	D -3	-	50‡
3	D -3	D -3	80§
4	D -9, -6, -3	-	10
5	D -9, -6, -3	D -9, -6, -3	25‡
6	D -9, -6, -3	D -3	32‡
7	-	D -3	12
8	-	D -9, -6, -3	14

*BALB/c male mice (6-8 wk old) were treated i.p. with MVE-2 (25 mg/kg) or indomethacin (6 mg/kg) at the days (D) indicated and sacrificed on day 0 for natural killer cell assay.
†Average of two separate experiments.
‡$\underline{P} = < 0.01$
§$\underline{P} = < 0.001$, compared to nontreated control.

It has been previously reported that PGE inhibits NK cell activity (2, 3). The results in the present study would indicate that the depression, or lack of NK response, could be due to the induction of PGE following multiple treatments with MVE-2.

4. DISCUSSION

The results presented indicate that after in vitro exposure to several BRMs, hM and mMϕ are stimulated to release PGE. Of the several BRMs tested: four are synthesized chemicals with quite different structures (poly ICLC, MVE-2, Azimexon, BM 41.332), one is a bacterial extract (LPS), and two are types of IFNs (murine and human). The poly ICLC and MVE-2 polymers and LPS are reported to induce IFN (23). Azimexon and BM 41.332 induce comparatively very low titers of IFN in mice (unpublished observations).

LPS, poly ICLC, BM 41.332 and murine IFN were found to be the more effective and consistent inducers of PGE by mMϕ and mBMC, while LPS and poly ICLC were the most effective inducers of significant levels of PGE by hM and hBMC. LPS has previously been reported to stimulate PGE production by mMϕ (5, 14), while poly IC has previously only been studied in regard to its ability to stimulate PGE production by human fibroblasts (29).

Since the most active agents stimulating the release of PGE from mMϕ, mBMC, hM and hBMC (LPS and poly ICLC) are known inducers of IFN, it is tempting to speculate that IFN was the proximal mediator for the observed effect. The response achieved with mMϕ treated with murine α,β IFN would be consistent with this possibility, but the results achieved with hM would seem to rule out this direct correlation. In contrast to the levels of PGE released by hM with poly ICLC and LPS, human α or β IFN did not stimulate any detectable release of PGE. Human monocytes were less sensitive to BRMs in regard to the amount of PGE released. The difference in their sensitivity may be due to several factors, e.g., species difference, a peculiarity of elutriated monocytes or the difference in stage of cell differentiation between human peripheral blood monocytes and resident peritoneal mMϕ. Human IFN has been reported to delay or inhibit the maturation of hM to Mϕ in vitro (30) as well as blocking granulopoietic differentiation (31). However, hM did respond best to LPS and poly ICLC as did the mMϕ.

Our observations indicate that PGE production by mMϕ and hM reaches plateau level within 24 h. Culture supernatants of mMϕ incubated with LPS were reported to contain maximum levels of PGE at 4 h and remain at these levels at 24 h (5). The "peak" time of PGE_2 production for peritoneal exudate cells from mice was reported to occur at 5 d after BCG inoculation (32). Results of the present study show that PGE production and release by mMϕ do not exceed those levels attained at 24 h. The plateau of PGE concentration did not increase with low PGE inducers during the longer incubation periods. With mMϕ, the magnitude or response to the BRMs was LPS > αβIFN > poly ICLC > BM 41.332. This lack of further release of PGE after 24 h indicates that the mMϕ have lost their capacity to produce and/or release PGE. When mMϕ previously exposed to LPS for 24 h were washed free of LPS and supernatant containing released PGE and reincubated with poly ICLC for an additional 24 h, no further release of PGE was detected. The same results were obtained when poly ICLC was employed first and then followed by LPS (unpublished observations). These results would indicate further that mMϕs are refractory to further PGE production and/or release. Possible explanations for this lack of further release of PGE could be that the in vitro conditions are not satisfactory for sustaining the metabolic function of the mMϕ or that the brief period of production and release of PGE may be an intrinsic biologic function of mMϕ.

Resident peritoneal mMϕ exposed to BRMs in vitro become cytolytic to tumor target cells (33). Addition of PGE to in vitro IFN activated mMϕ markedly inhibited their tumoricidal activity (4, 34, 35). Recent reports confirm the observation that the acquisition and loss of cytolytic activity of resident peritoneal mMϕ are time dependent and related to the production of PGE by the mMϕ (5, 36). LPS-stimulated mMϕ remained cytolytic to tumor target cells for 12 to 16 h, and then their activity decreased. This decrease was attributable to the release and accumulation of PGE. The released PGE did not act by blocking the development of mMϕ cytolytic activity but limited the activity via a feedback inhibition mechanism (5, 34, 35, 36).

Each of the BRMs which induced the secretion of elevated PGE levels by mMϕ (poly ICLC, mαβIFN, BM 41.332, LPS, Table 4) also stimulated GM-CSF secretion. The simultaneous secretion of GM-CSF and PGE by mMϕ suggests that both mediators have the same cellular origin; however, it is possible that two subsets of Mϕ may be responsible for the secretion of either PGE or GM-CSF alone, as proposed elsewhere (20). Our data indicate that secretion of the two factors is not directly linked, since inhibition of PGE secretion by indomethacin did not block secretion of GM-CSF. These data also indicate that PGE, at levels present in the supernatants, did not interfere with GM-CFU-C growth in culture. This is further supported by data (Table 5) showing that only high levels of PGE significantly inhibited GM-CFU-C growth in vitro. Such high PGE levels, however, were not reached in our GM-CSF assay. These findings are in contrast with reports showing an inhibitory effect of PGE on GM-CFU-C growth in vitro at PGE levels > 10^{-9} M (21, 37). While our results at high concentrations of PGE support the hypothesis that PGE may have a negative feedback effect on GM-CFU-C growth (21, 37) one may question the biological importance of these data since pharmacologic and not physiologic levels (38, 39) were required for such an in vitro inhibitory effect. It cannot, however, be excluded that the required inhibitory PGE levels are locally achievable in vivo.

Inhibition of mouse NK cells by PGE (2, 40, 41) and human NK cells by PGE_2 (42) has been reported previously. PGE_2 released by mMϕ in vivo has also been implicated in the inhibition of NK cell activity (32, 43). The role of PGE_2 in the augmentation of NK cell activity was studied by administering PGE cyclooxygenase inhibitors, indomethacin and aspirin, before BCG inoculation in mice (32). Such treatment resulted in reduced PGE_2 production and potentiated NK cell augmentation. The mMϕ was shown to regulate NK activity in the BCG-inoculated mice by secreting PGE_2. We show similar results when indomethacin was administered concomitantly with multiple treatments of MVE-2. The augmented NK cell activity in the hyporesponsive mice, mediated by the indomethacin treatment, supports the hypothesis that PGE_2 production, probably by the highly activated mMϕ, led to the decrease in NK cell activity.

The mMϕ appears to play a central role in the regulation of both mMϕ and NK cell activity since it appears to be the sole or major source of both the inhibitory PGE and stimulatory factors, such as IFN (44). Such opposing factors may be involved in the regulation of Mϕ and NK cell activity in the host treated with BRMs. Examining BRMs for their capacity to induce the production and secretion of PGE by Mϕs in vitro and in vivo would be of value in identifying a biological activity which could exert an antagonistic effect on other activities stimulated by BRMs such as NK cell augmentation or Mϕ cytolytic activity.

REFERENCES

1. Goldyne ME, Stobo JD: Immunoregulatory role of prostaglandin and related lipids. CRC Crit Rev Immunol (2): 189, 1982.

2. Brunda MJ, Herberman RB, Holden HT: Inhibition of murine natural killer cell activty by prostaglandins. J Immunol (124): 2682, 1980.

3. Koren HS, Anderson SJ, Fischer DG, Copeland CS, Jensen PJ: Regulation of human natural killing. I. The role of monocytes, interferon and prostaglandins. J Immunol (127): 2007, 1981.

4. Schultz RM, Stoychkov JN, Pavlidis N, Chirigos MA, Olkowski ZL: Role of E-type prostaglandins in the regulation of interferon-treated macrophage cytotoxic activity. J Reticuloendothel Soc (26): 93, 1979.

5. Taffet SM, Russell SW: Macrophage-mediated tumor cell killing: Regulation of expression of cytolytic activity by prostaglandin E. J Immunol (126): 424, 1981.

6. Wieder KJ, Webb DR: The effect of prostaglandin metabolism on immunoglobulin and antibody production in naive and educated whole spleen cells. Prostaglandin Med (7): 79, 1981.

7. Baker PE, Fahey JV, Munck A: Prostaglandin inhibition of T-cell proliferation is mediated at two levels. Cell Immunol (61): 52, 1981.

8. Goodwin JS, Messner RP, Peake GT: Prostaglandin suppression of mitogen-stimulated lymphocytes in vitro. J Clin Invest (62): 753, 1978.

9. Leung KH, Mihich E: Effects of prostaglandins on the development of cell-mediated immunity in culture and on the cytolytic activity of in vivo generated effector cells. Int J Immunopharmacol (4): 205, 1982.

10. Pelus LM, Broxmeyer HE, Kurland JI, Moore MAS: Regulation of macrophage and granulocyte proliferation. J Exp Med (150): 277, 1979.

11. Trevisani A, Ferretti E, Capuzzo A, Tomasi V: Elevated levels of prostaglandin E_2 in Yoshida hepatoma and the inhibition of tumor growth by non-steroidal anti-inflammatory drugs. Br J Cancer (41): 341, 1980.

12. Kurland JI, Bockman R: Prostaglandin E production by human blood monocytes and mouse peritoneal macrophages. J Exp Med (147): 952, 1978.

13. Bonney RJ, Wightman PD, Davies P, Sadowski SJ, Kuehl FA, Humes JL: Regulation of prostaglandin synthesis and of the selective release of lysosomal hydrolases by mouse peritoneal macrophages. Biochem J (176): 433, 1978.

14. Wahl LM, Rosenthal DL, Glode LM, Sandberg AL, Mergenhagen SE: Defective prostaglandin synthesis by C3H/HeJ mouse macrophages stimulated with endotoxin preparations. Infect Immun (23): 8, 1979.

15. Chirigos MA, Mitchell M, Mastrangelo MJ, Krim M: Mediation of Cellular Immuity in Cancer by Immune Modifiers. Raven Press, New York, 1981.

16. Stevenson HC, Katz P, Wright DG, Contreras TJ, Jemionek JF, Hartwig VM, Flor WJ, Fauci AS: Human blood monocytes: Characterization of negatively selected human monocytes and their suspension cell culture derivatives. Scand J Immunol (14): 1, 1981.

17. Schlick E, Friedberg KD: Bone marrow cells of mice under the influence of low lead dose. Arch Toxicol (49): 227, 1982.

18. Steel LK, Kaliner M: Prostaglandin-generating factor of anaphylaxis. J Biol Chem (256): 12692, 1981.

19. Steel LK, Platshon L, Kaliner M: Prostaglandin generation by human and guinea pig lung tissue. Comparison of parenchymal and airway responses. J Allergy Clin Immunol (64): 387, 1979.

20. Pelus LM, Broxmeyer HE, DeSousa M, Moore MAS: Heterogeneity among resident murine peritoneal macrophages: Separation and functional characterization of monocytoid cells producing granulocyte-macrophage colony-stimulating (GM-CSF) and responding to regulation by lactoferrin. J Immunol (126): 1016, 1981.

21. Pelus LM, Broxmeyer HE, Kurland JI, Moore MAS: Regulation of macrophage and granulocyte proliferation. Specificities of prostaglandin E and lactoferrin. J Exp Med (150): 277, 1979.

22. Herberman RB, Nunn ME, Lavrin DH: Natural cytotoxic reactivity of mouse lymphoid cells against syngeneic and allogeneic tumors. Int J Cancer (16): 216, 1975.

23. Chirigos MA, Mastrangelo MJ: Immunorestoration by chemicals. In: Mihich E (ed) Immunological approaches to cancer therapeutics. John Wiley & Sons, New York, 1982, pp 191-239.

24. Herberman RB, Brunda MJ, Cannon GB, Djeu JY, Nunn ME, Jett JR, Ortaldo JR, Reynolds C, Riccardi C, Santoni A. In: Hersh EM et al. (eds) Augmenting agents in cancer therapy. Raven Press, New York, 1981, pp 253-265.

25. Maluish AE, Ortaldo JR, Conlon JC, Sherwin SA, Leavitt R, Strong DM, Weirnik P, Oldham RK, Herberman RB: Depression of natural killer cytotoxicity after in vivo administration of recombinant leukocyte interferon. J Immunol (131): 503, 1983.

26. Bruley-Rosset M, Rappaport H: Natural killer cell activity and spontaneous lymphoma development. Effect of single and multiple injections of interferon in young and aged C57BL/6 mice. Int J Cancer (31): 381, 1983.

27. Piccoli M, Saito T, Chirigos MA: Biomodal effects of MVE-2 on cytotoxic activity of natural killer cell and macrophage tumoricidal activities. Int J Immunopharmacol, 1984, in press.

28. Bartocci A, Papademetriou V, Chirigos MA: Enhanced macrophage and natural killer cell antitumor activity by various molecular weight maleic anydride divinyl ethers. J Immunopharmacol (2): 49, 1980.

29. Yaron M, Yaron I, Wiletzki C, Zor U: Interrelationship between stimulation of prostaglandin E and hyaluronate production by poly (I) poly (C) and interferon in synovial fibroblast culture. Arthritis Rheum (21): 694, 1978.

30. Lee SH, Epstein LB: Reversible inhibition by interferon of the maturation of human peripheral blood monocytes to macrophages. Cell Immunol (50): 177, 1980.

31. Verma DS, Spitzer G, Zander AR, Gutterman JV, McCredie KB, Dicke KA, Johnston DA: Human leukocyte interferon preparation-mediated block of granulopoietic differentiation in vitro. Exp Hematol (9): 63, 1981.

32. Tracey DE, Adkinson, Jr. NF: Prostaglandin synthesis inhibitors potentiate the BCG-induced augmentation of natural killer cell activity. J Immunol (125): 136, 1980.

33. Schultz RM, Papamatheakis JD, Chirigos MA. In: Chirigos MA (ed) Immune modulation and control of neoplasia by adjuvant therapy. Raven Press, New York, 1978, pp 459.

34. Schultz RM, Pavlidis NA, Stylos WA, Chirigos MA: Regulation of macrophage tumoricidal function: A role for prostaglandins of the E series. Science (202): 320, 1978.

35. Schultz RM, Jackson WT. In: Chirigos MA, Mitchell M, Mastrangelo MJ, Krim M (eds) Mediation of cellular immunity in cancer by immune modifiers. Raven Press, New York, 1981, pp 89.

36. Shaw JO, Russell SW, Printz MP, Skidgel RA: Macrophage-mediated tumor cell killing: A lack of dependence on the cyclooxygenase pathway of prostaglandin synthesis. J Immunol (123): 50, 1979.

37. Kurland JI, Hadden JW, Moore MAS: Role of cyclic nucleotides in the proliferation of committed granulocyte-macrophage progenitor cells. Cancer Res (37): 4534, 1977.

38. Jaffee BM, Behrman HR, Parker CW: Radioimmunoassay measurement of prostaglandin E, A and F in human plasma. J Clin Invest (52): 398, 1973.

39. Berenbaum MC, Cope WA, Bundick RV: Synergistic effect of cortisol and prostaglandin E_2 on the PHA response. Clin Exp Immunol (26): 534, 1976.

40. Henney CS, Tracey DE, Durdik JM, Klimpel G: Natural killer cells: In vitro and in vivo. Am J Path (93): 459, 1978.

41. Roder JC, Klein M: Target-effector interactions in the natural killer cell system. II. Modulation by cyclic nucleotides. J Immunol (123): 2785, 1979.

42. Droller MJ, Schneider MV, Pearlmann P: A possible role for prostaglandins in the inhibition of natural and antibody-dependent cell-mediated cytotoxicity against tumor cells. Cell Immunol (39): 165, 1978.

43. Tracey DE, Davis JW, Taggart MT, Silberman SL: Modulation of natural killer cell activity by interferons and prostaglandins. Afr J Clin Exp Immunol (3): 19, 1982.

44. Unanue ER: The regulation of lymphocyte functions by the macrophage. Immunol Rev (40): 227, 1978.

ACKNOWLEDGMENTS

K.H. was supported by Boehringer GmbH, Mannheim, FRG, and E.S. was supported by Deutsche Krebshilfe, Bonn, FRG.

Chapter 9

THE ROLE OF ARACHIDONIC ACID METABOLITES IN THE REGULATION OF NEUTROPHIL FUNCTION

H.M. KORCHAK and S.B. ABRAMSON

1. INTRODUCTION

Acute inflammation is provoked by a wide variety of mediators. These mediators may affect vascular tone and permeability (e.g. histamine, serotonin), stimulate peripheral pain receptors (e.g. bradykinin), as well as attract and activate inflammatory cells (e.g. complement components, platelet activating factor). The release of mediators from such inflammatory cells (including metabolites of arachidonic acid, lysosomal proteases and oxygen-derived products such as superoxide anion) promote the permanent destructive tissue damage characteristic of the acute inflammatory response.

It is generally accepted that products of arachidonic acid are involved in inflammation. Their precise role is complex and includes the modulation of neutrophil activation.

2. NEUTROPHILS

2.1 Release of mediators: stimulus-response coupling

The mature human neutrophil is highly specialized for its primary function, the phagocytosis, killing and digestion of microorganisms. Appropriately opsonized particles elicit cell- cell aggregation, ingestion, killing and degranulation responses. In conditions where these functions are defective, the host is subject to recurrent infections. Neutrophils are also commonly found at sites of inflammation, and through release of their granule contents, active oxygen species and arachidonate derivatives (5HETE, leukotriene B_4), are probably responsible for the development and amplification of the inflammatory response and its associated tissue destruction (1).

The release of granule contents and superoxide anion normally occurs into the closed phagocytic vacuole. Closure of the phagocytic vacuole can be prevented by the addition of cytochalasin B. Under these conditions the neutrophil is converted into a secretory cell. The physiology of the neutrophil can therefore be treated in a fashion analogous to the secretory responses of endocrine and exocrine organs.

Ligand binding to surface receptors (Fc, concanavalin A, chemotactic peptide, complement components C5a and C3b, and phorbol myristate acetate receptors), as well as perturbation of the membrane with the calcium ionophore A23187, have been shown to initiate superoxide anion generation, degranulation and aggregation responses. The events that follow ligand binding and lead to the release of these inflammatory mediators have been termed "stimulus-response coupling." Involved are complex movements of divalent cations, the generation of cyclic AMP and protein phosphorylation. The modulation of neutrophil function by arachidonate metabolites appears to result from their effects on these critical intermediary events. To better elucidate the effects of these compounds on neutrophil function the details of stimulus-response coupling will first be reviewed.

2.2 Cell activation sequence: calcium and cyclic AMP

2.2.1 Cell responses to ligands. The neutrophil is a professional phagocyte which normally secretes lysosomal contents and superoxide anions (O_2^-) into the phagocytic vacuole during particle ingestion. The binding of specific ligands such as immune complexes, chemotactic peptides, the complement component C5a, the lectin concanavalin A and phorbol myristate acetate (PMA) to the plasmalemma, initiates activation of the neutrophil. When phagocytic vacuole closure is prevented by treating the cell with the fungal metabolite cytochalasin B, the granule contents and O_2^- are secreted into the medium where they can readily be monitored. In this way secretion can be quantitatively compared with the extent of other cellular changes. The stimuli that trigger O_2^- generation and degranulation also initiate cell-cell aggregation which can by measured in the presence or absence of cytochalasin B.

2.2.2 Calcium and signalling. In the neutrophil, calcium appears to play a role as a second messenger, as it does in other systems (2,3). The calcium ionophore A23187 can bypass the receptor ligand interaction causing the influx of extracellular calcium which is followed by degranulation, superoxide anion generation and aggregation (4,5). In addition, it has been shown that calcium depleted neutrophils can be induced to secrete lysozyme by re-exposure to calcium. The relative roles of intra- and extracellular calcium in the activated neutrophil have been assessed (6,7). Removal of Ca^{2+}, either by omission from the medium, or by addition of EGTA, reduced but did not entirely abolish the generation of superoxide anion, aggregation or degranulation in response to a variety of stimuli. In contrast, the agent 8-(N,N-diethyl amino)-octyl-3,4,5 -trimethoxybenzoate hydrochloride (TMB8), which is a reported antagonist of intracellular mobilization in muscle (8), caused a dose dependent inhibition of f-Met-Leu-Phe induced degranulation, aggregation and superoxide anion generation by cytochalasin B treated human neutrophils (6,7). Such studies indicate that the mobilization of intracellular Ca^{2+} is the rate limiting step for neutrophil activation while the entrance of extracellular Ca^{2+} is essential for optimal neutrophil function.

Cytoplasmic Ca^{2+} has been proposed as a key regulator of cell activation. The fluorescent, highly selective Ca^{2+} indicator, Quin2 can be trapped inside cells, where it serves as a rapid and sensitive indicator of changes in cytoplasmic free Ca^{2+}. Using this probe, Tsien et al. have been able to demonstrate a rapid rise in cytoplasmic free calcium in f-Met-Leu-Phe activated cells (9). There was no measurable lag period. We have confirmed these results (10) and have also demonstrated that Con A and IgG activated neutrophils demonstrate a rise in cytosolic free calcium. The rise in cytosolic free calcium was one of the earliest measurable responses in both f-Met-Leu-Phe, IgG and Con A activated cells, lending support to the hypothesis that increments in cytosolic free calcium serve as a signal to activate the subsequent physiological responses. However a rise in free cytoplasmic calcium is not an absolute requirement for neutrophil activation, since when neutrophils were activated with the tumor promoter PMA, no increment in cytosolic free Ca^{2+} was observed (10). Nevertheless, superoxide anion generation, release of specific granules and aggregation were activated by PMA. It has been suggested that PMA may bypass the calcium requiring segment of the activation sequence by directly activating a protein kinase C (10,11).

In order for calcium to play a regulatory role in neutrophil function, its intracellular concentration must be strictly regulated. Consequently, one or more pools of cell-associated calcium must exist from which calcium can be mobilized by cell stimulation and into which ionic calcium can be sequestered. Although the sites at which calcium is sequestered and from which it can be mobilized have been identified in skeletal muscle, the sites of its sequestration have not been as well defined in non-muscle cells. Changes in membrane associated calcium can be monitored using the probe chlortetracycline which forms highly fluorescent complexes with membrane Ca^{2+} or Mg^{2+}. The fluorescence of CTC-labelled neutrophils decreases promptly upon exposure to a variety of stimuli (12,13). The prompt kinetics of this response, observed 2-5 secs after stimulation, suggests that one of the earliest events in neutrophil activation is the release of membrane-bound calcium. The pool of membrane associated calcium monitored by CTC appears not to be the source of the elevated cytosolic calcium monitored by Quin2.

2.2.3 Cyclic nucleotides and signalling. Cyclic AMP is a "second messenger" in many secretory systems. In the neutrophil, however, exogenous cAMP is not sufficient to activate the secretory response. Cyclic AMP, but not cGMP, is transiently elevated in activated neutrophils (14-18), a process that is greatly amplified in the presence of the prostaglandins PGE_1 and PGI_2. Herlin et al (15) have shown that exposure of human neutrophils to latex provoked a rapid increase in cAMP levels. This increase was prompt (maximal within 15 sec) and brief. These workers suggested that the brief rise in cAMP might have a regulatory role in glycogen metabolism (15). Further studies have demonstrated a rapid transient rise in cAMP levels in neutrophils exposed to chemotactic stimuli (14-18). Similar rises in cAMP levels were also noted with immune complexes and A23187 activated neutrophils (14), the rise in cAMP occurred after a discernible lag period but preceded the onset of superoxide anion generation, aggregation and degranulation. However, Con A and phorbol myristate actetate, which are good stimuli for O_2^- generation as well as the release of specific but not azurophil granule release, provoked no change in cAMP levels (19). Thus only "complete secretagogues" (e.g. f-Met-Leu-Phe, immune complexes, A23187 which elicit degranulation of both azurophil and specific granules) caused a cAMP elevation; "incomplete" stimuli (e.g. con A and phorbol myristate acetate which elicit only specific granule secretion) did not cause any change in cAMP levels (19). Further evidence that functional responses of neutrophils are independent of changes in cAMP was obtained by Simchowitz et al (20). In the presence of the adenyl cyclase inhibitor, 9-(tetrahydro-2-furyl) adenine, the increments in cAMP usually observed in f-Met-Leu-Phe and A23187 activated neutrophils were completely inhibited (20), whereas degranulation and superoxide anion generation were unaffected, additional evidence that functional responses are not dependent on changes in cAMP levels. It has been well documented that cAMP, and agents (such as beta agonists) which elevate intracellular levels of cAMP diminish both degranulation and other cellular responses of neutrophils (21) suggesting a role for cyclic nucleotides in the regulation of neutrophil activation. In the activated neutrophil, cAMP appears to act as a modulator but not as a signal for cell function.

Cyclic AMP appears to act as a feedback inhibitor in neutrophils, since agents that elevate cAMP also inhibit secretion (21). It is of interest that the negative feedback mediator cAMP has been shown to inhibit the enhanced calcium permeability accompanying activation, indicating the existence of a complex system of regulatory loops "fine tuning" the activity of the cell. Intracellular calcium and cAMP appear to be regulated in an interdependent fashion (22). Controls exerted by cyclic nucleotides operate within the context of the cell's ionic network, shifts of intra- and extra-cellular ions act to modulate such processes as endocytosis and exocytosis.

2.2.4 Protein phosphorylation. Phosphorylation of proteins is involved in the regulation of the intracellular activities of numerous cell types by external stimuli. A cAMP sensitive protein kinase has been shown in the cytosol of human neutrophils (23). In human neutrophils activated by a variety of stimuli, such as PMA, opsonized zymosan, f-Met-Leu-Phe and digitonin (24) enhanced phosphorylation of four protein bands was observed. Similarly, in rabbit neutrophils, addition of f-Met-Leu-Phe, C5a or LTB4 enhanced phosphorylation of a number of proteins. Both cAMP and phospholipid sensitive protein kinase activities were observed with these stimuli (23). It is of interest that the phorbol diester receptor copurifies with protein kinase C in rat brains (25). Such an activity might explain why PMA can bypass the need for elevated cytosolic calcium in the activation sequence.

2.3 Phospholipid turnover and the arachidonic acid cascade

Stimulated neutrophils remodel their phospholipids to release arachidonic acid.

In many tissues (26,27), including neutrophils (28-33), the addition of hormones or other ligands that stimulate Ca^{2+} entry, results in an increased breakdown of phosphatidyl inositol (PI) to diglyceride (DG), phosphorylation of the DG to phosphatidic acid (PA) and finally resynthesis of PI. This sequence of events is initiated by the action of a phospholipase C. It has been

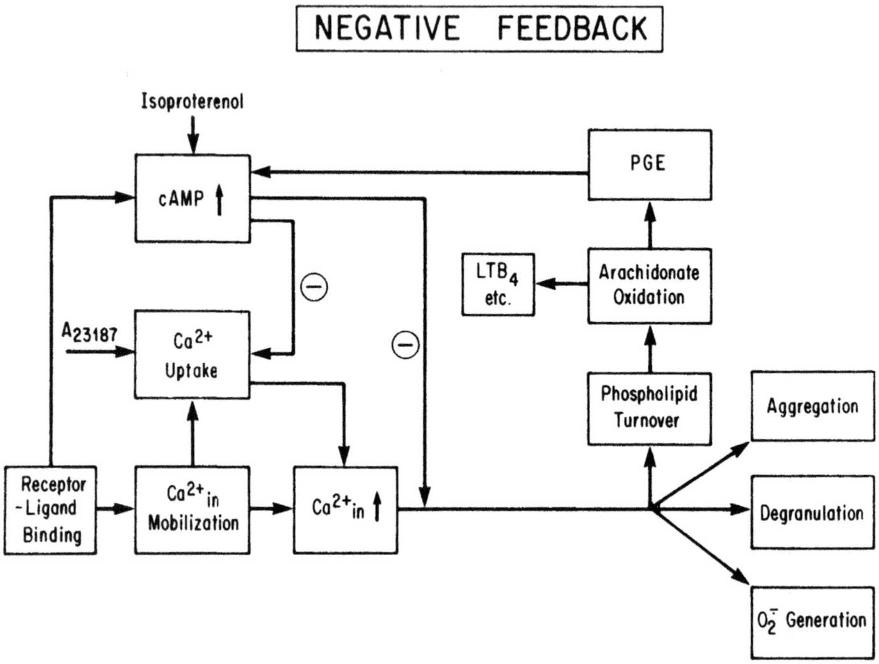

FIGURE 1. Schema of events associated with the activation of the neutrophil. Negative feedback control exerted by stable prostaglandins. See text for details.

proposed that the PI breakdown induced by ligand-receptor interaction might be directly involved in controlling calcium entry into the cell. In addition, arachidonic acid may be released by cleavage from the diglyceride or from the phosphatidic acid. Alternatively, arachidonic acid may be released, principally from phosphatidyl choline, by the action of a phospholipase A_2. Stimulated neutrophils actively generate oxygenated arachidonic acid derivatives, principally by the 5 lipoxygenase pathway (see below). Thus arachidonate derivatives, produced during the remodeling of membrane phospholipids, are available locally to modulate cell function.

3. PROSTAGLANDINS

3.1. Prostaglandins as modulators of inflammation

Prostaglandins may act as mediators of inflammation due to their capacity to provoke the classical signs of inflammation: heat, swelling, erythema and pain. It is well established that PGE_2 and PGI_2 are potent vasodilators and capable of acting synergistically with histamine to increase vascular permeability. Similarly these compounds enhance bradykinin-induced pain. When injected intrathecally arachidonic acid and PGE_2 provoke fever. High levels of PGE_2 have been reported in the joint fluids from patients with inflammatory arthritis (1), with subsequent lowering of these levels following treatment with NSAID (34). Samples of rheumatoid synovium in culture have been shown to produce large amounts of PGE_2 (35). PGE's furthermore have been shown to have significant bone resorbing activity (36).

In certain experimental models, however, prostaglandins have been shown to <u>inhibit</u> inflammatory cells.

Each of the cells of acute and chronic inflammation (platelets, neutrophils, macrophages and lymphocytes) are able to transform arachidonic acid into biologically active derivatives. Arachidonic acid may be oxidized via the cyclooxygenase pathway, which was found by Vane to be inhibited by aspirin and many other nonsteroidal anti-inflammatory drugs. The first intermediate of arachidonate transformation is an endoperoxide (PGG_2) in which molecular oxygen has been added. Subsequently the PGG_2 is transformed to PGH with the liberation of an oxygen-derived free radical. These endoperoxides have a very short half life in biological fluids and are rapidly transformed into stable prostaglandins, prostacyclin and thromboxane. Neutrophils activated by a physiological stimuli such as f-Met-Leu-Phe, however, do not generate significant quantities of stable prostaglandins. Nevertheless, prostaglandins produced by other cell types (e.g. macrophages, endothelial cells) are available to modulate neutrophil function.

3.2 Effect of prostaglandins on neutrophil function

Stable prostaglandins inhibit the in vitro activation of neutrophils. Prostaglandins of the E and I series, when added to neutrophils, inhibit the release of granule contents as well as the generation of O_2^- (2,37-39). This inhibition of cell responses occurred when neutrophils were activated with f-Met-Leu-Phe, opsonized particles (zymosan) or A23187. Prostaglandins were shown to possess inhibitory activity at low, physiological levels of 5 nM. Recent work has demonstrated that the prostaglandin analog 15alpha-11-deoxy-8-azaPGE_1 also inhibited the respiratory burst of neutrophils while the analogue 15 epi-11deoxy-8-azaPGE_1 did not exert this effect (40). The inhibitory action of prostaglandins was not confined to degranulation and O_2^- generation, since prostaglandins were also shown to inhibit cell-cell aggregation in response to f-Met-Leu-Phe and immune complexes (41,42).

3.3 Coupling of prostaglandin receptors to adenylate cyclase

Prostaglandins of the E and I series work via receptors on the cell membrane that are linked to the adenylate cyclase system, thereby raising intracellular cAMP (37). In the presence of the phosphodiesterase inhibitor theophylline, which inhibits the breakdown of cAMP, the cAMP levels elicited by prostaglandins were enhanced. Concentrations of prostaglandin E_1 and prostaglandin I_2 which were sufficient to inhibit lysosomal enzyme release, produced sustained levels of cAMP in resting cells. Stimulation of prostaglandin pretreated cells evoked very large increases in cAMP, 8 to 10-fold basal level. Thus exposure to prostaglandins "primes" the cells such that the usual modest increments in cAMP accompanying activation are greatly magnified into higher, probably inhibitory levels. In support of such a hypothesis, it was found that the phosphodiesterase inhibitor theophylline, which enhances the resulting cAMP levels, also enhance the inhibitory efficacy of the prostaglandins. A physiological level of PGE (5 nM) was shown to inhibit O_2^- generation and aggregation; this effect was enhanced by the presence of theophylline.

In contrast to the findings in f-Met-Leu-Phe activated neutrophils, the O_2^- generation activated by PMA was only moderately inhibited by PGE_1 (38). Since PMA does not elicit elevated cAMP levels, these findings constitute further support for the hypothesis that prostaglandins inhibit neutrophil functions via a cAMP dependent mechanism.

3.4 Prostaglandins and calcium mobilization

The classical second messengers proposed for a variety of different cell types are calcium and cAMP. Elevation of cAMP has previously been shown to modulate some calcium movements during neutrophil activation. It therefore seemed possible that prostaglandins could inhibit neutrophil activation via an effect on calcium movements, and furthermore that this proposed effect would be dependent on cAMP.

As previously discussed, the fluorescent probes chlortetracycline and Quin2 can be used to measure the mobilization of calcium from two different intracellular pools. Quin2 monitors changes in free cytosolic calcium while CTC is thought to monitor changes in membrane (plasmalemma) associated Ca.

3.5 Prostaglandins, cAMP and cytosolic calcium levels

Neutrophils activated with f-Met-Leu-Phe show a rapid elevation cytosolic calcium to a level of approximately 1 uM. This rapid elevation in cytosolic calcium is followed by a slow recovery phase to resting levels of cytosolic calcium. Neither physiological (nanomolar) levels or pharmacologial (micromolar) levels of PGE were found to inhibit either the rise in cytosolic calcium, or the recovery process. (43,44). Addition of 500 uM theophylline to PGE_1 did not affect the peak of the response. PGE_1 therefore has no effect on the Quin2 fluorescence response (i.e., peak cytosolic calcium), nor was the rate of recovery affected. Therefore, the profound inhibition of neutrophil responses such as lysosomal enzyme release, superoxide anion generation, and aggregation by PGE cannot be due to an inability of PGE treated cells to raise cytosolic Ca levels.

3.6 Prostaglandins, cAMP and chlortetracycline fluorescence changes

Chlortetracycline (CTC) is commonly used as a probe for membrane associated calcium. Loss of CTC fluorescence occurs immediately (i.e. within one second), subsequent to the addition of stimulus, a loss that is thought to monitor the release of a "trigger pool" of calcium associated with secretion. The fluorescence loss in response to f-Met-Leu-Phe was highly sensitive to the presence of PGE; inhibition was demonstrated at PGE doses as low as 5 nM (44,45). Furthermore, the inhibition was enhanced in the presence of theophylline, suggesting synergy between PGE_1 and theophylline and implicating cAMP in the inhibitory effect of PGE_1 on the CTC response. Indeed, addition of dibutyryl cAMP was shown to inhibit CTC fluorescence changes.

In contrast to the findings in f-Met-Leu-Phe activated neutrophils, Con A and the tumor promotor phorbol myristate acetate (PMA) do not elicit a rise in cAMP in prostaglandin pre-treated cells. The CTC fluorescence response of cells stimulated by ligands such as Con A and PMA was only minimally affected by the presence of PGE. This effect was not enhanced by the presence of theophylline. Compared to their effect on f-Met-Leu-Phe stimulated cells, prostaglandins only modestly affect the CTC response of Con A and PMA stimulated cells. The profound inhibition of the CTC response by prostaglandins is only seen in cells in which there is an associated rise in cAMP (e.g., in FMLP stimulated cells). Thus, elevated cAMP appears necessary for the inhibition of the CTC response by PGE_1.

Inhibition of aggregation and superoxide anion generation took place at both high and low concentrations of PGE_1 in f-Met-Leu-Phe stimulated cells. The inhibition of these two responses cannot be due to defective elevation of cytosolic calcium. However, these functional changes are associated with defective mobilization of plasmalemmal calcium as measured by CTC. Therefore, PGE_1, acting via the negative modulator cAMP inhibits neutrophil function by inhibiting mobilization of a discrete pool of plasmalemmal calcium.

4. LEUKOTRIENES

4.1 Products of the neutrophil.

In stimulated human neutrophils, the enzymatic oxygenation of liberated arachidonic acid occurs predominantly through the lipoxygenase pathway (46). The activation of the cell's 5-lipoxygenase produces a series of monohydroxylated eicosatetraenoic acids (mono-HETEs), some of which exhibit chemoattractant properties as

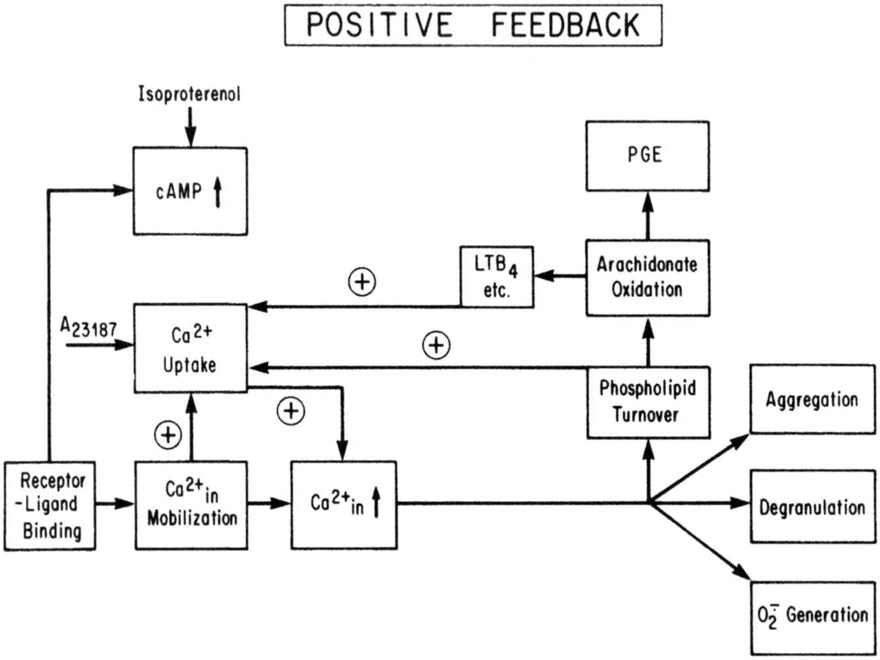

FIGURE 2. Positive amplification of neutrophil activation by leukotrienes. See text for details.

described below. The mono-HETE, 5-hydroxy eicosatetraenoic acid, may be further converted to the unstable epoxide leukotriene A_4 which serves as a precursor to leukotriene B_4 (LTB_4). The formation of LTB_4 from LTA_4 occurs either through enzymatic hydroxylation or through non-enzymatic oxygenation (47). The recovered lipoxygenase products depend in part on the stimulus employed. When cells are activated with calcium ionophores, such as A23187, or with crystalline monosodium urate, LTB_4 is the main product generated (48,49). When the chemoattractant f-met-leu-phe is used, recoverable LTB_4 is reduced whereas later inactive metabolites of LTB_4 including the biologically inactive omega-OH and COOH derivatives constitute the principle recoverable products (49). In addition to LTB_4, activated neutrophils generate sulfide peptide leuktrienes such as LTC_4, LTD_4 and LTE_4 which are broken down extracellularly by a myeloperoxidase - H_2O_2-Cl^- dependent system (50).

The lipoxygenase products of arachidonic acid generated by the activated neutrophil are increasingly appreciated as important mediators of acute inflammation. While they exhibit effects on the microcirculation, such as enhancing vascular permeability, perhaps the most critical role of these compounds is their capacity to attract and activate other neutrophils.

4.2. Effects of monoHETEs on neutrophil function

Quantitatively, 5-HETE is the most abundant arachidonate metabolite produced by the activated neutrophil (46). Both this compound and the related product of platelet activation, 12-HETE, have been demonstrated to be chemoattractants for other neutrophils. Furthermore, work by Stenson and Parker has demonstrated that both 5-HETE and 12-HETE induce degranulation of specific, but not azurophilic, granules of these cells (51). Lysosomal enzyme release is achieved at 5- to 10 uM concentrations somewhat higher than the concentrations optimal for chemotaxis (51). The work of Goetzl et al (52,53) demonstrated that optimally chemotactic concentration of 5-HETE (1-2 ug/ml) increased the expression of neutrophil receptors for C3b. These same concentrations of 5-HETE not only failed to provoke superoxide production by neutrophils but actually caused a modest reduction (33%) in the generation of this free radical (52).

4.3. Effects of leukotriene B_4 on neutrophil function

4.3.1. In vitro. While produced by the neutrophil in lesser quantity than 5-HETE, LTB_4 (5S,12R diHETE), is the most potent inflammatory derivative of the lipoxygenase pathway. It is approximately 100-fold more potent a chemoattractant than the mono-HETEs (54). Effective at picogram quantities, LTB_4 is equivalent to FMLP and C5a as a chemoattractant (55-59). Unlike the mono-HETEs, LTB_4 is a complete secretagogue causing degranulation of both specific and azurophil granules (47). Indeed, LTB_4 at concentrations of 10^{-8}M is capable of initiating the full host of neutrophil responses, including mobilization of membrane associated calcium, aggregation, superoxide anion generation and degranulation (47).

4.3.2. In vivo. Work in animal models has corroborated the inflammatory potential of LTB_4 in vivo. Injection of LTB_4 into the pleural or peritoneal cavity is followed rapidly by the accumulation of large numbers of neutrophils (55). Injected into the anterior chamber of a rabbit eye as little as 25 nanograms of LTB_4 provokes as intense inflammatory response. When injected intravenously into hamsters, LTB_4 provokes increased margination of neutrophils (60). Co-administration sub-cutaneously of both LTB_4 and PGE_2 or bradykinin was synergistic in provoking an inflammatory response with increased vascular permeability (54,61,62).

4.3.3. Mechanism of LTB_4 induced neutrophil activation. Work by several laboratories (52,63) has suggested that LTB_4 binds to human neutrophils via specific cell surface receptors. In studies by Kreisle and Parker (63), binding ^3H-LTB_4 was demonstrated at nanomolar concentrations, (i.e. concentrations at which cellular responses occur), with saturation occurring at 10 X 10^{-6} molar. Binding was blocked by (^{14}C) LTB_4 but not by

(3H)-FMLP. Stereospecificity was demonstrated by diminished binding of 6-trans and 12-epi-6-trans-isomers of LTB_4, an observation consistent with the known lesser biologic activity of these compounds. These studies, demonstrating saturability and specificity are consistent with the presence of a specific receptor for LTB_4 on the neutrophil surface.

Work by Serhan (47,48), alternatively, has suggested that LTB_4 may also serve as an ionophore in the neutrophil by initiating the translocation of calcium. These studies made use of artificial lipid bilayers, liposomes, which are devoid of cell surface receptors (47). Experiments demonstrated that, like the calcium ionophore A23187, LTB_4 could promote the permselective translocation of calcium across intact lipid bilayers. As has been the case in other biologic systems, there was a requirement for the "cis" configuration of LTB_4 as "trans" isomers were inactive. In related studies, the effect of LTB_4 and known calcium ionophores on neutrophil functions was compared. In each instance (aggregation, superoxide anion generation, degranulation, and decrements of chlortetracycline fluorescence) LTB_4 behaved comparably to A23187. It was proposed that LTB_4 might activate the neutrophil via two mechanisms, able to engage specific receptors and serve as a calcium ionophore in neutrophils. Since full neutrophil responsiveness was not achieved until concentrations of LTB_4 exceeded 10^{-8} M they suggested that at concentrations less than 10^{-8} M LTB_4 interacts with its receptor whereas at higher concentrations it behaved as a calcium ionophore, bypassing receptors and directly causing a rise in intracellular calcium (48).

Whether by ligand-receptor binding or by the direct promotion of calcium translocation, the ability of LTB_4 (a neutrophil product), to activate the neutrophil, likely serves as an important amplifier of the inflammatory response.

4.4 Interactions of lipoxygenase and cyclooxygenase products

When released extracellularly products of both the lipoxygenase and cyclooxygenase pathways are postulated to contribute to the development of the inflammatory response. They may act synergistically as has been demonstrated for the capacity of PGE_1 and LTB_4 to increase vascular permeability. However, it is also apparent from the preceding discussion that the stable prostaglandins and LTB_4 exert opposing effects on neutrophil function. PGE_1, PGE_2 and PGI_2, for example, effectively inhibit calcium mobilization, adherence, aggregation, superoxide generation and lysosomal enzyme release by the stimulated neutrophil. These effects are believed to be due to the ability of these agents to increase levels of cyclic AMP which renders the cell less responsive to subsequent stimulation. It is not unexpected therefore that a recent report by Ham et al has demonstrated that, at physiologic concentrations (5×10^{-7} M) PGE_1 and PGE_2 also totally suppressed the release of LTB_4 from FMLP stimulated rat peritoneal neutrophils (64) Since LTB_4 increases neutrophil adherence, these authors speculate that the production of prostaglandins by endothelial cells will suppress adhesion of neutrophils to vascular endothelium by inhibiting LTB_4 production. We have observed furthermore that LTB_4-induced activation of the neutrophil (aggregation, superoxide generation) is significantly depressed in the presence of PGE_1. One would anticipate therefore that PGE_1 would dampen the inflammatory response both by decreasing the production of LTB_4 as well as by rendering other neutrophils less responsive to that LTB_4 produced.

Thus, products of arachidonate metabolism have complex and, at times, opposing effects on the activation of the neutrophil. Their production at sites of inflammation may serve to modulate the intensity of the phlogistic response.

Acknowledgements

This investigation was supported by Grant Number AI 18676, awarded by the National Institutes of Health to Dr. Korchak. Dr. Abramson is a Fellow of the Arthritis Foundation.

References

1. Trang LE: Prostaglandins and Inflammation. Seminars Arth. & Rheum 9: 153-190, 1980

2. Douglas WW: Involvement of calcium in exocytosis and the exocytosis vesiculation sequence. Biochem. Soc. Symp. (39):1-28, 1974.

3. Putney JE: Stimulus-permeability coupling: role of calcium in the receptor regulation of membrane permeability. Pharmacol. Rev. (30): 209-245, 1979

4. Goldstein IM, Horn JK, Kaplan HB, Weissmann G: Calcium induced lysozyme secretion from human polymorphonuclear leukocytes. Biochem. Biophys. Res. Comm. (60):807-812, 1974.

5. O'Flaherty JT, Showell HJ, Becker EL, Ward PA: Substances which activate neutrophils. Mechanism of action. Am. J. Path. (92):155-166, 1978.

6. Smith RJ, Wierenga W, Iden S: Characteristics of N-formyl-methionyl-leucyl-phenylalanine as an inducer of lysosomal enzyme release from human neutrophils. Inflamm. (4):73-88, 1980

7. Smolen JE, Korchak HM, Weissmann G: The roles of extracellular and intracellular calcium in lysosomal enzyme release and superoxide anion generation by human neutrophils. Biochim. Biophys. Acta (677):512-520, 1981.

8. Malagodi MH, Chiou CY: Pharmacological evaluation of a new calcium antagonist 8-(N,N-diethylamino)--octyl-3,4,5-trimethoxybenzoate hydrochloride (TMB-8): Studies in smooth muscle. Eur. J. Pharmacol. (27):25-33, 1974.

9. Pozzan T, Lew DP, Wollheim CB, Tsien RY: Is cytosolic ionized calcium regulating neutrophil activation? Science (221):1413-1415, 1983

10. Korchak HM, Vienne K, Rutherford LE, Wilkenfeld, C, Finkelstein MC, Weissmann G: Stimulus response coupling in the human neutrophil II Temporal analysis of changes in

cytosolic calcium and calcium efflux. J. Biol. Chem. (259),4076-4082, 1984

11. Sando JJ, Young MC: Identification of high-affinity phorbol ester receptor in cytosol of EL-4 thymoma cells: requirement for calcium, magnesium and phospholipids. Proc. Natl. Acad. Sci. USA (80):2642-2646, 1983

12. Smolen JE, Weissmann G: The effect of various stimuli and calcium antagonists on the fluorescence response of chlortetracycline-loaded human neutrophils. Biochim. Biophys. Acta (720):172-180, 1982.

13. Naccache PH, Showell HJ, Becker EL, Sha'afi RI: Involvement of membrane calcium in the responce of rabbit neutrophils to chemotactic factors as evidenced by the fluorescence of chlortetracycline. J. Cell Biol. (83):179-186, 1979.

14. Smolen JE, Korchak HM, Weissmann G: Increased levels of cyclic adenosine-3',5'-monophosphate in human polymorphonuclear leukocytes after surface stimulation. J. Clin. Invest. (65):1077-1085, 1980.

15. Herlin T, Petersen CS, Esmann V: The role of calcium and cyclic adenosine-3',5'-monophosphate in the regulation of glycogen metabolism in phagocytosing human polymorphonuclear leukocytes. Biochim. Biophys. Acta (542):63-76, 1978.

16. Jackowski S, Sha'afi RI: Response of adenosine cyclic-3',5'-monophosphate level in rabbit neutrophils to the chemotactic peptide formylmethionyl-leucyl-phenylalanine. Molec. Pharmacol. (16):473-481, 1979.

17. Simchowitz L, Fischbein LC, Spilberg I, Atkinson JP: Induction of a transient elevation in intracellular levels of adenosine 3',5'-cyclic monophosphate by chemotactic factors: An early event in human neutrophil activation. J. Immunol. (124):1482-14911, 1980.

18. Keller HU, Gerisch G, Wissler J: A transient rise in cyclic AMP levels following chemotactic stimulation of neutrophil granulocytes. Cell Biol. Internat. Reports (3):759-765, 1979.

19. Smolen JE, Weissmann G: Stimuli which provoke secretion of azurophil enzymes from human neutrophils induce increments in adenosine cyclic 3'-5'monophosphate. Biochim. Biophys. Acta (672):197-206, 1981.

20. Simchowitz L, Spilberg I, Atkinson JP: Evidence that the functional responses of human neutrophils occur independently of transient elevations in cAMP levels. Fed. Proc. (42): 1080, 1983.

21. Zurier RB, Weissmann G, Hoffstein S, Kammerman S, Tai H: Mechanisms of lysosomal enzyme release from human leukocytes II. Effects of cAMP and cGMP, autonomic agonists and agents which affect microtubule function. J. Clin. Invest. (43):297-309, 1974.

22. Rasmussen H. and Goodman DBP: Relationships between calcium and cyclic nucleotides in cell activation. Physiol. Rev. (57):421, 1977.

23. Huang C-K, Hill Jr J, Mackin WM, Bormann BJ, Becker EL: Effects of chemotactic factors on the protein phosphorylation of rabbit peritoneal neutrophils. Fed. Proc. (92):1080, 1983.

24. Andrews PC, Babior BM: Endogenous protein phosphorylation by resting and activated human neutrophils. Blood (61):333-340, 1983.

25. Niedel JE, Kuhn LJ, Vandenbark GR: Phorbol diester receptor copurifies with protein kinase C Proc. Natl. Acad. Sci. USA (80):36-40, 1983.

26. Kirk CJ: Ligand-stimulated inositol lipid metabolism in the liver: Relationship to receptor function. Cell Calcium (3): 399-412, 1982.

27. Berridge MJ, Fain JN: Inhibition of phosphatidyl inositol synthesis and the inactivation of calcium entry after prolonged exposure of the blowfly salivary gland to 5-hydroxytryptamine. Biochem. J. (178): 58-69, 1979.

28. Karnovsky M L, Shafer AW, Cagan RH, Graham RC, Karnovsky MJ, Glass EA, Saito K: Membrane function and metabolism in phagocytic cells. Trans. N. Y. Acad. Sci. (28): 778-787, 1966.

29. Sostry PS, Hokin LE: Studies on the role of phospholipids in phagocytosis. J. Biol. Chem. (241): 3354-3361, 1966.

30. Tou J-S, Stjernholm RL: Stimulation of the incorporation of ^{32}Pi and myo(2^{3}H)-inositol into the phosphoinositides in polymorphonuclear leukocytes during phagocytosis. Arch. Biochem. (160): 487-494, 1974.

31. Tou J-S: Modulation of ^{32}Pi incorporation into phospholipids of polymorphonuclear leukocytes by ionophore A23187. Biochim. Biophys. Acta (531): 167-178, 1978.

32. Cockcroft S, Bennett JP, Gomperts BD: F-Met-Leu-Phe-induced phosphatidyl inositol turnover in rabbit neutrophils is dependent on extracellular calcium. FEBS Letters (110): 115-118, 1980.

33. Serhan C, Korchak HM, Broekman J, Smolen JE, Marcus A, Weissmann G: Phosphatidyl inositol breakdown and phosphatidic acid accumulation in stimulated human neutrophils: Relationship to calcium mobilization and calcium uptake. Biochim. Biophys. Acta (In Press)

34. Bombardieri S et al: The synovial prostaglandin system in chronic inflammatory arthritis: Differential effects of steroidal and non-steroidal anti-inflammatory drugs. Br. J. Pharm. (73):893-901, 1981.

35. Dayer JM, Krane SM et al: Production of collagenase and prostaglandins by isolated adherent

rheumatoid synovial cells. Proc. Natl Acad. Sci. USA (73):945-949, 1976.

36. Robinson DR et al: Prostaglandin-stimulated bone resorption by rheumatoid synovial. J. Clin. Invest. (56):1181, 1975.

37. Weissmann G, Smolen JE, Korchak H: Prostaglandins and Inflammation: Receptor/cyclase Coupling as an Explanation of why PGEs and PGI_2 Inhibit Functions of Inflammatory Cells" in Advances in Prostaglandins and Thromboxane Research, Vol. 8, B. Samuelsson, B., Ramwell, P.W. and Paoletti, R. eds, Raven Press, New York, pp 1637-1653, 1980.

38. Fantone JC, Kinnes DA: Prostaglandin E_1 and Prostaglandin I_2 modulation of superoxide production by human neutrophils. Biochem. Biophys. Res. Comm. (113): 506-512, 1983.

39. Wong K, Freund K: Inhibition of the n-formyl-methionyl-leucyl-phenylalanine induced respiratory burst in human neutrophils by adrenergic agonists and prostaglandins of the E series Can. J. Physiol. Pharmacol. (59): 915-92L, 1981.

40. Spisani S, Vicenzi E, Traniello S, Pollini G P., Barco A: Synthetic prostaglandin analogue: In vitro studies on human neutrophils. Immunopharmacol (4): 323-330, 1982.

41. O'Flaherty JT, Kreutzer DL, Ward PA: Effect of Prostaglandins E_1, E_2 and F_{2a} on Neutrophil aggregation Prostaglandins (17): 201-209, 1979.

42. Camussi G, Tetta C, Bussolino F, Cappio FC, Coda R, Masera C, Segoloni G: Mediators of immune-complex -induced aggregation of polymorphonuclear neutrophils II. Platelet-activating factor as the effector substances of immune-induced aggregation. Int. Archs. Allergy Appl. Immun. (64): 25-41, 1981.

43. Lew PD, Dayer J-M, Wollheim CB, Pozzan T: Effect of leukotriene B_4, prostaglandin E_2 and arachidonic acid on cytosolic-free calcium in human neutrophils. FEBS Letts. (166): 44-48, 1984.

44. Abramson S, Korchak H, Kimmel S, Roberts C, Wilkenfeld C, Haines K, Rich A, Rider L, Weissmann G: The cellular effects of nonsteroidal antiinflammatory drugs (NSAID) cannot be due to inhibition of prostaglandin (PG) release. Arth. Rheum. (27):S22, 1984.

45. Smolen JE: The fluorescence response of chlortetracycline-loaded human neutrophils is modulated by prostaglandin E_1, but not by cyclic nucleotides. FEBS Letts. (163): 119-123, 1983.

46. Stenson WF, Parker CW: Metabolism of arachidonic acid in ionophore-stimulated neutrophils. J. Clin. Invest. (64):1457-1465, 1979.

47. Serhan CN, Smolen JE, Korchak HM, Weissmann G: Leukotriene B_4 is a complete secretagogue in human

neutrophils: Ca2+ translocation in liposome and kinetics of neutrophil activation. In: Samuelsson B, Paoletti R, Ramwell P (ed) Adv. Prostaglandin and Thromboxane Res. Raven Press, New York, 1983, pp 53-63.

48. Serhan CN, Fridovich J, Goetzl EJ, Dunham PB, Weissmann G: Leukotriene B_4 and phosphatidic acid are calcium ionophores. J. Biol. Chem. (257):4746-4752, 1982.

49. Serhan CN, Lundberg U, Weissmann G, Samuelsson B: Formation of leukotrienes and hydroxy acids by human neutrophils and platelets exposed to monosodium urate. Prostaglandins (27):563-581, 1984.

50. Less CW, Lewis K, Austen F, Corey EJ: Oxidative inactivation of the sulfidopeptide leukotrienes by human polymorphonuclear leukocytes (PMNs). Fed. Proc. (42): 1080-1084, 1983.

51. Stenson WF, Parker CW: Monohydroxyeicosatetraenoic acids (HETEs) induce degranulation of human neutrophils. J. Immunol. (124):2100-2104, 1980.

52. Goetzl EJ, Brash AR, Tauber AI, Oates JA, Hubbard WC: Modulation of human neutrophil function by monohydroxyeicosatetraenoic acids. Immunology 39:491-501, 1980.

53. Goetzl EJ, Sun FF: Generation of unique monohydroxyeicosatetraenoic acids from arachidonic acid by human neutrophils. J. Exp. Med. 150:460-

54. Bray MA, Ford-Hutchinson AW, Smith MJH: Leukotriene B_4: Biosynthesis and biologic activity. In: SRS-A and Leukotrienes (Piper, PJ, ed.) Chichester, Research Studies Press, Inc., pp 253-270, 1981.

55. Smith MJH, Ford-Hutchinson AW, Bray MA: Leukotriene B: A potential mediator of inflammation. J. Pharm. Pharmacol. (32):517-518, 1982.

56. Higgs GA, Bax CMP, Moncada S: Inflammatory properties of lipoxygenase products and the effects of indomethacin and BW 755 c on prostaglandin production, leukocyte migration and plasma exudation in rabbit Skin. In. Adv. Prostaglandin Thromboxane Leukotriene Res. Raven Press, New York, (9), pp 331-339, 1982.

57. Malmsten CL, Palmblad J, Uden A-M, Radmark O Engstedt L, Samuelsson B: Leukotriene B_4: A highly potent stereospecific factor stimulating migration of polymorphonuclear leukocytes of different species. Prostaglandins (20):411-418, 1980.

58. Bhattacherjee P, Hammond B, Salmon JA, Stepney P, Eakins KE: Chemotactic response to some arachidonic acid lipoxygenase products in the rabbit eye. Eur. J. Pharmacol. (73):21-28, 1981.

59. Ford-Hutchinson AW, Bray MA, Doig MV, Shipley ME, Smith MJ: Leukotriene B_4, a potent chemokinetic and aggregating substance released from polymorphonuclear leukocytes. Nature (286):264-265, 1980.

60. Dahlen S-E, Bjork J, Hedqvist P, Arfors K-E, Hammarstrom S, Lindgren J-A, Samuelsson B: Leukotrienes promote plasma leakage and leukocyte adhesion in postcapillary venules: In vivo effects with relevance to the acute inflammatory response. Proc. Natl. Acad. Sci. USA (78):3887-3891, 1981

61. Bray MA, Cunningham FM, Ford-Hutchinson AW, Smith MJH: Leukotriene B_4: A mediator of vascular permeability. Br. J. Pharmacol. (72):483-486, 1981.

62. Williams TJ, Jose PJ, Wedmore CV, Peck MJ, Forest MJ: Mechanisms underlying inflammatory edema: The importance of synergism between prostaglandins, leukotrienes and complement derived peptides. In: Adv. Prostaglandin and Thromboxane Res., Raven Press, New York, 11:33-37, 1983.

63. Kreisle R, Parker C: Specific binding of leukotriene B_4 to a receptor on human polymorphonuclear leukocytes. J. Exp. Med. (157):628-641, 1983.

64. Ham EA, Soderman DD, Zanetti ME, Dougherty HW, McCauley E, Kuehl FA: Inhibition by prostaglandins of leukotriene B_4 release from activated neutrophils. Proc. Natl. Acad. Sci. USA (80):4349-4353, 1983.

INDEX

GPSR Compliance

The European Union's (EU) General Product Safety Regulation (GPSR) is a set of rules that requires consumer products to be safe and our obligations to ensure this.

If you have any concerns about our products, you can contact us on ProductSafety@springernature.com

In case Publisher is established outside the EU, the EU authorized representative is:

Springer Nature Customer Service Center GmbH
Europaplatz 3
69115 Heidelberg, Germany

Batch number: 10755292

Printed by Printforce, the Netherlands